Families as Allies in Treatment of the Mentally Ill: New Directions for Mental Health Professionals

Families as Allies in Treatment of the Mentally Ill: New Directions for Mental Health Professionals

Edited by

Harriet P. Lefley, Ph.D.

*Professor, Department of Psychiatry, University of Miami
School of Medicine, Miami, Florida*

Dale L. Johnson, Ph.D.

*Professor, Department of Psychology, University of Houston,
Houston, Texas*

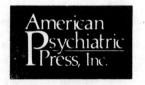

American Psychiatric Press, Inc.

1400 K Street, N.W.
Washington, DC 20005

Note: The authors have worked to ensure that all information in this book concerning drug dosages, schedules, and routes of administration is accurate as of the time of publication and consistent with standards set by the U.S. Food and Drug Administration and the general medical community. As medical research and practice advance, however, therapeutic standards may change. For this reason and because human and mechanical errors sometimes occur, we recommend that readers follow the advice of a physician who is directly involved in their care or the care of a member of their family.

Books published by the American Psychiatric Press, Inc., represent the views and opinions of the individual authors and do not necessarily represent the policies and opinions of the Press or the American Psychiatric Association.

The paper used in this publication meets the minimum requirements of the American National Standard for Information Sciences—Permanence of Paper for Printed Library Materials, ANSI Z39.48-1984. ∞

Library of Congress Cataloging-in-Publication Data

Families as allies in treatment of the mentally ill / edited by Harriet P. Leafley, Dale L. Johnson.—1st ed.
    p.   cm.
Consists mostly of expanded and updated versions of papers originally presented at the National Forum on Educating Mental Health Professionals to Work with Families of the Long-Term Mentally Ill, held in Rockville, Md. in Feb. 1986, organized as a joint effort of the National Institutes of Health and the National Alliance for the Mentally Ill.
Includes bibliographical references.
ISBN 0-88048-298-2
    1. Mentally ill—Family relationships—Congresses. 2. Mental health personnel—Congresses. 3. Mentally ill—Rehabilitation—Congresses. I. Lefley, Harriet P. II. Johnson, Dale L., 1929–   . III. National Forum on Educating Mental Health Professionals to Work with Families of the Long-Term Mentally Ill (1986: Rockville, Md.) IV. National Institute of Mental Health (U.S.) V. National Alliance for the Mentally Ill (U.S.)
    [DNLM: 1. Mental Disorders—rehabilitation—congresses. 2. Professional-Family Relations—congresses. 3. Psychiatry—education—congresses. WM 29 M549]
RC455.4.F3M46   1989
616.89′023—dc20
DNLM/DLC   LC-89-17778
for Library of Congress   CIP

Contents

Contributors ix

Foreword xiii
   Shervert Frazier, M.D.

Introduction: On Educating Mental Health
Professionals to Work With Families of the Long-Term
Mentally Ill xv
   Harriet P. Lefley, Ph.D.

Part I

Overview of Issues

1 **A Historical Perspective on Family-Provider
Relationships** 3
   Kenneth G. Terkelsen, M.D.

   Commentary to Chapter 1
   **Continuing Problems Between Mental Health
   Professionals and Families of the Mentally Ill** 23
   H. Richard Lamb, M.D.

2 **The Family's Experience of Living With Mental
Illness** 31
   Dale L. Johnson, Ph.D.

   Commentary to Chapter 2
   Can the Family Literature Be Integrated? 65
   William R. McFarlane, M.D.

3 **The Social Context of Helping Families** 77
   Agnes B. Hatfield, Ph.D.

   Commentary to Chapter 3
   The Disabled Family 91
   Leona L. Bachrach, Ph.D.

4 **Family-Provider Relationships: Charting a New Course** 99
   Kayla F. Bernheim, Ph.D.

Commentary to Chapter 4
Care of the Chronically Mentally Ill: Is It Honorable Work? 115
   Carol M. Anderson, Ph.D.

5 **Research Directions for a New Conceptualization of Families** 127
   Harriet P. Lefley, Ph.D.

Commentary to Chapter 5
How Goes the Battle? 163
   Samuel J. Keith, M.D.
   H. Alice Lowery, Ph.D.

Part II

Models for Educating Professionals

6 **Ethical and Legal Considerations for Interviewing Families of the Seriously Mentally Ill** 173
   Evelyn McElroy, R.N., Ph.D.

Commentary to Chapter 6
Informed Consent, Confidentiality, and Contracting 195
   Leroy Spaniol, Ph.D.

7 **Promoting Institutional Acceptance of New Paradigms: An Approach to the Professional Schools** 201
   Gerda Cohen, A.C.S.W.
   Kenneth G. Terkelsen, M.D.

Commentary to Chapter 7
Teaching Psychiatrists About the Family's Experience 217
   Christian C. Beels, M.D.

8 **A Curriculum Guide for Fieldwork in Chronic Mental Illness** 223
   Mona Wasow, A.C.S.W.

Commentary to Chapter 8
**Competence-Based Training of Psychiatric
Practitioners in the Rehabilitation of the
Chronically Mentally Ill** 241
  Timothy G. Kuehnel, Ph.D.
  Robert Paul Liberman, M.D.

9 **Functioning of Relatives and Patients Facing
Severe Mental Illness** 255
  Shirley Glynn, Ph.D.
  Robert Paul Liberman, M.D.

Commentary to Chapter 9
**Guidelines for Working With Families of the
Chronically Mentally Ill** 267
  Christine McGill, Ph.D.

Index 279

Contributors

Carol M. Anderson, Ph.D.
Professor, Western Psychiatric Institute and Clinic,
Pittsburgh, Pennsylvania

Leona L. Bachrach, Ph.D.
Professor, Maryland Psychiatric Research Center, University
of Maryland School of Medicine, Catonsville, Maryland

Christian C. Beels, M.D.
Professor, New York State Psychiatric Institute, New York,
New York

Kayla F. Bernheim, Ph.D.
Clinical Psychologist, Livingston County Counseling Services,
Mt. Morris, New York

Gerda Cohen, A.C.S.W.
Psychotherapist in private practice, Scarborough, New York

Shervert Frazier, M.D.
General Director/Psychiatrist-in-Chief, McLean Hospital,
Belmont, Massachusetts

Shirley Glynn, Ph.D.
Clinical Psychologist, Camarillo UCLA Research Center,
Camarillo, California

Agnes B. Hatfield, Ph.D.
Professor Emeritus, Department of Human Development,
University of Maryland, College Park, Maryland

Dale L. Johnson, Ph.D.
Professor, Department of Psychology, University of Houston, Houston, Texas

Samuel J. Keith, M.D.
Deputy Director, Division of Clinical Research, and Associate Director for Schizophrenia Programs, National Institute of Mental Health, Rockville, Maryland

Timothy G. Kuehnel, Ph.D.
Assistant Professor, UCLA School of Medicine, West Los Angeles VA Medical Center, Los Angeles, California

H. Richard Lamb, M.D.
Professor, Department of Psychiatry, University of Southern California School of Medicine, Los Angeles, California

Harriet P. Lefley, Ph.D.
Professor, Department of Psychiatry, University of Miami School of Medicine, Miami, Florida

Robert Paul Liberman, M.D.
Professor, University of California, Los Angeles, West Los Angeles VA Medical Center, Los Angeles, California

H. Alice Lowery, Ph.D.
Chief, Psychosocial Treatment and Rehabilitation Program, Schizophrenia Research Branch, National Institute of Mental Health, Rockville, Maryland

Evelyn McElroy, R.N., Ph.D.
Associate Professor, University of Maryland School of Nursing, Baltimore, Maryland

William R. McFarlane, M.D.
Professor, New York State Psychiatric Institute, New York, New York

Christine McGill, Ph.D.
Assistant Clinical Professor, Department of Psychiatry, University of California, San Francisco, California

Leroy Spaniol, Ph.D.
Editor, *Psychosocial Rehabilitation Journal*, Center for Rehabilitation Research and Training in Mental Health, Boston University, Boston, Massachusetts

Kenneth G. Terkelsen, M.D.
Assistant Clinical Professor and Director, Day Treatment,
Department of Psychiatry, Cornell University Medical
College, Mt. Vernon, New York

Mona Wasow, A.C.S.W.
Clinical Professor, University of Wisconsin School of Social
Work, Madison, Wisconsin

Foreword

In February 1986, during my tenure as director, the National Institute of Mental Health (NIMH) was pleased to support an event of potentially historic significance for clinical training. The National Forum on Educating Mental Health Professionals to Work With Families of the Long-Term Mentally Ill brought together a group of people representing unique and valuable perspectives. The conference was organized by members of the Curriculum and Training Committee of the National Alliance for the Mentally Ill (NAMI), a committee composed primarily of mental health professionals involved in graduate education or clinical training who have experienced major mental illness in members of their own families. The task of this committee has been to educate colleagues on the experiential impact of mental illness on the family and to demonstrate ways in which professionals can provide more sensitive and effective services that families perceive as truly responsive to their needs. These NAMI committee members invited a group of colleagues to engage in a dialogue on theoretical and empirical issues that have affected the relationships of families and mental health professionals. In addition to the NAMI participants, the group included prominent academicians, researchers, and clinicians who have devoted a good part of their professional lives to the needs of the chronically mentally ill population. The purpose of the meeting was to develop dialogue, and hopefully consensus, on issues involving theory, technology, and social policy that might lead to new directions in contemporary treatment and clinical training of future professionals.

This book represents an update and expansion of some of the formal papers and responses that formed the core of this conference. Unfortunately, the richness and depth of the discussion and the synergistic exchange of ideas cannot be captured in a bound volume of papers. There was a remarkably high level of enthusiasm among all participants, and a shared feeling that new ground was being broken in understanding and improving the relationships between families of the mentally ill and the practitioners who serve their loved ones. All agreed that the conference was a notable beginning for what continues to be an ongoing discussion of issues. The meeting subsequently led to the involvement of other prominent educators and family theorists, including leaders in the field, in an ongoing dialogue on new directions in clinical training and research.

Involvement of knowledgeable consumers in the planning process for service delivery and in the training of present and future practitioners have been avowed goals of NIMH. This volume is clearly a step in that direction. We hope that the dialogue will continue to flourish and, by so doing, to generate ever-improved levels of service for the chronically mentally ill and their families.

Shervert Frazier, M.D.

Introduction: On Educating Mental Health Professionals to Work With Families of the Long-term Mentally Ill

Most scientists recognize that the broad course of history will ultimately confirm, modify, or discredit their theories. Indeed, the long process of hypothesis testing, multiple replications, and rigorous investigations of spin-offs or of serendipitous findings is the essence of the scientific endeavor. Establishing a sound knowledge base may involve many years of refuting old truths and developing and testing alternative models.

Individuals who are personally involved with the issues being studied, however, cannot afford to wait for history to catch up with their needs. Their lives, and those of their loved ones, are vitally affected by inadequate or wrongful theories and their applications. Because they are in a state of immediate pain, they need a research base, and informed interpretations of available data, that will lead to technologies that they perceive as most reasonable and experience as most beneficial given the current state of the art.

Surveys of families of the mentally ill indicate considerable dissatisfaction with many of the unconfirmed technologies currently applied to themselves and their loved ones (Hatfield 1983; Holden and Lewine 1982; Spaniol et al. 1984). This dissatisfaction is also reflected among mental health professionals who have family members with major long-term mental illnesses (Lefley 1987). It is the families of this category of patients—those with severely disabling schizophrenias, major affective disorders, and other long-term psychotic conditions—who constitute the target group of our efforts.

The chapters in this book focus on developing new models for conceptualizing the interrelationships among professionals, patients, and their families. In former years, professionals related to such families only through their patients, primarily in terms of assumed pathogenesis. In the interests of the therapeutic alliance, therapists had as little interaction as possible with family members. In the contemporary climate of family therapy, professionals have as much interaction as possible with family members, relating to them as unidentified patients and as objects of therapeutic change. Family members have indicated that they do not appreciate the restricted range of either role. In educating clinicians of the future, a new role must be conceptualized for families of the mentally ill.

This book evolved from the National Forum on Educating Mental Health Professionals to Work With Families of the Long-Term Mentally Ill, organized as a joint effort of the National Institute of Mental Health and the National Alliance for the Mentally Ill (NAMI). The forum was convened with the long-range objective of modifying clinical education so that families of the mentally ill will be viewed and will perceive themselves as being viewed as allies rather than as adversaries by new generations of professionals.

When we consider the range of theoretical and pragmatic questions that have been raised in the literature, we may want to consider a core question in terms of four components. Given our present state of knowledge, what is the best way of conceptualizing the role of families of the mentally ill with respect to 1) the patient, 2) family members, 3) mental health professionals and the provider system, and 4) society as a whole? We might consider a sample of the following:

1. Focusing on the patient:
   • What is our current thinking about families and pathogenesis?
   • Should the patient's treatment modalities involve the family? If so, which models are most beneficial?
   • What are the best ways to train families in patient management and care giving?
   • What is the appropriate role of families in symptom control or tertiary prevention?
2. Considering the impact of mental illness on family members:
   • What should clinicians know about objective and subjective family burden?
   • To what extent do the legal and provider systems contribute to family burden?
   • Are families of the mentally ill a priori dysfunctional? Can we make a statement about the concept of family deviance?

- What are some of the coping strategies and strengths of families in dealing with mental illness?
3. On relations of families and the provider system:
   - What are the reciprocal perceptions of mental health professionals and families? Is there a continuity of past and present attitudes and behaviors?
   - What are the appropriate modes of communication between professionals and families of patients?
   - Which are the most profitable areas of family-provider collaboration? Is there a role for families in clinical training?
   - What is the preferred role for families in service delivery or in the continuum of care?
4. On relations of families and the larger society:
   - Are there general cultural factors that stigmatize families and affect their self-perception? What are the operative factors in changing these views?
   - What are the appropriate roles of government (local, state, federal) and families in providing care for the disabled?
   - How do legal protections of patients impact on families and on the patient-family relationship?
   - What are the most profitable directions for family advocacy with respect to research and services?

The discussion papers at this conference dealt with a historical overview of the conceptualization of family roles, the realities of experiencing mental illness in the family, contemporary social policy issues, the relationships between providers and families, and research questions that need to be resolved. One of the major research issues deals with whether families of persons with long-term psychotic disorders will continue to be considered deviant, and the scope and function of this perception by the professional community. Questions were raised regarding the unique, cumulative stressors that may affect the behavior of family members, particularly in their interactions with mental health professionals; possible iatrogenesis of family "psychopathology" in various contexts, both distal and proximal; and the extent to which behavioral patterns and family-patient and family-provider relationships are a product of cultural values and belief systems.

The papers that emerged from this forum raise critical issues that require resolution. Is it necessary for clinicians to anticipate and work with deficiencies rather than strengths in families in order to have something to offer? Why is there so much criticism of the concepts of expressed emotion and psychoeducational interventions, when they seem to provide the very services that patients' relatives have been demanding from providers—information and behavior management techniques? Yet problems are inherent in interventions that seem to focus on families alone both as toxins and as remedial resources (Hatfield 1987). Is the therapeutic modality a political statement? What ethical and legal problems are raised in the interactions of professionals and families? What are the most fertile research directions for resolving some of these questions, for reconceptualizing the family's role in mental illness, and for determining the most beneficial mode of family-provider relationships?

Assuming that we are able to attain consensus on some or most of these questions, how can we best take our knowledge to the training institutions? Can we enable clinicians to view families as groups of individuals coping with inordinate pain, stressors, and life disruptions, rather than as malfunctioning systems contributing to the patient's psychopathology? Can we teach them to view families as an asset rather than a liability, as a resource rather than an antagonist to the therapeutic process? Can we thus enable new generations of clinicians to develop new models of working collaboratively with families, through provision of professional expertise, consultation and liaison with advocacy groups, training, and partnership in resource development? Can we teach them also to enhance their own technologies by learning from families about human strengths, coping strategies, and learned techniques for prevention of relapse? Finally, what are the best ways of promoting institutional change and acceptance of new paradigms by mental health professionals?

This book contains contributions from a number of professionals who have personal knowledge of the effects of long-term mental illness on the family. Individuals with this dual vantage point have a vital interest in these issues, beyond the typical academic investments of ideology and career. Our purpose, however, is not to substitute one set of dogmas for another, but rather to accelerate the processes of discovery and change. We expect to find a diversity of opinions, agendas, and expectancies among NAMI members as well as among others who are expert in issues regarding the long-term mentally ill. The contributed chapters and their commentaries address these issues by suggesting fertile areas for new models of service, research, and training. We believe the time may be ready for more salutary concepts of family role and for training future clinicians in new ways of perceiving and interacting with the families of their patients.

Harriet P. Lefley, Ph.D.

REFERENCES

Hatfield AB: What families want of family therapists, in Family Therapy in Schizophrenia. Edited by McFarlane WR. New York, Guilford, 1983, pp 41–65

Hatfield AB: The expressed emotion theory: why families object. Hosp Community Psychiatry 38:341, 1987

Holden DF, Lewine RRJ: How families evaluate mental health professionals, resources, and effects of illness. Schizophr Bull 8:626–633, 1982

Lefley HP: Impact of mental illness in families of mental health professionals. J Nerv Ment Dis 175:613–619, 1987

Spaniol L, Jung H, Zipple AM, et al: Families as a central resource in the rehabilitation of the severely psychiatrically disabled: report of a national survey. Unpublished report, Boston, MA, Boston University, Center for Rehabilitation Research and Training in Mental Health, 1984

Part I

Overview of Issues

A Historical Perspective on Family-Provider Relationships

Kenneth G. Terkelsen, M.D.

As the chronically mentally ill have been turned out of large institutions and placed in the communities of America, it has become apparent that collaboration among patients, their relatives, and their professional care givers is a fundamental prerequisite of stable and dignified community tenure. Yet, for a long time, relations between relatives and mental health professionals have been filled with so much tension that there is very little mutually acceptable common ground for that collaboration. Additionally, the focus of professional attention has remained on the mentally ill, even though one of the most dramatic effects of the move into the community has been a tangible increase in burden for other family members.

Those of us who are mental health professionals and have family members who are mentally ill are faced with the unique challenge of knowing both worlds. There is now an effort to replace animosity and mistrust with a mutual capacity for respect and collaboration. We believe that this new common ground will enable families and professionals to work for the benefit of the severely mentally ill living in America's communities without at the same time losing sight of the family's ongoing needs and adding to its burden through indifference and excessive care-giving expectations.

WHY A HISTORICAL PERSPECTIVE?

As I undertook this task, I was mindful of the complexity and tenacity of the forces involved in the current stalemate. One reason for this complexity is that we are two turns along the road, down a hill and around a bend from whence our predecessors of a century and a half ago fashioned an American approach to mental illness. Those early workers did not have the benefit of contemporary neuroscience with which to assess the validity of their theories. Rather, at a time of major societal transition, they were influenced by the face validity of ideas linking social deviance to social structure. In the current era, we may easily forget that their point of departure was an unprecedented determination to heal and that its effect on the medical enterprise of the ensuing 150 years derives largely from that determination.

My thesis in this chapter is that the negative relationships now in evidence between relatives of the mentally ill as a group and mental health professionals as a group are an unrecognized legacy of three historically powerful forces in American social thought. These forces had, in their time, profound effects on the arrangements of care of the mentally ill and incidentally on the relations between the mentally ill, their families, and the professional medical community. The effects have endured even though the social theories that set these arrangements in motion are at least partially eclipsed in the contemporary American intellectual climate. Specifically, many professional attitudes and practices that are now troublesome to family care givers are remnants of policies and practices that first took shape during the mid–nineteenth century as a part of the asylum approach to mental illness. These were in turn deepened and given a more problematic meaning due to the weight assigned to family experience in early twentieth century psychoanalytic ideas about the etiology of the psychoses and in treatment approaches that attempted to bring about changes in here-and-now family interaction. Finally, families were confounded by the efforts beginning in the 1950s to return the mentally ill home from hospitals and to discourage family efforts to seek long-term institutional care where such care had never been attempted.

I divide my discussion into five sections. First, I will review very briefly what is known about the emergence of the insane asylum as a treatment for mental illness. Second, I will review the psychoanalytic orientation toward the psychoses and its extension into family therapy. Third, I will look at the intellectual foundations of the deinstitutionalization movement. In each section, the central question is What did it mean for the family? Fourth, I will show how certain contemporary professional attitudes and institutional practices can be seen as remnants of each of these formerly popular treatments, outliving the intellectual microclimates in which they flourished. Finally, I will describe some aspects of what might optimally emerge as the norm for relations between families of the mentally ill and mental health providers in decades to come.

EVOLUTION OF ASYLUMS FOR THE INSANE IN THE UNITED STATES

Rothman (1971) has studied the development of asylums in the United States, showing that asylums for the care of the insane emerged in the United States during the first half of the nineteenth century at a time when similar institutions were evolving for related purposes in other deviant populations (e.g., orphanages for children, almshouses for the poor, and penitentiaries for criminals). At inception, the anticipated functions of these new institutions were twofold. Asylums would protect the mentally ill from the stresses of life in the open community. American society was undergoing massive dislocations during this era, placing new kinds of stress on all citizens. The presumption that these social stresses played a primary role in the etiology of mental illness was rising in popularity among lay and medical communities alike. Large institutions for the insane were expected to accord relief from those stresses, thereby halting the advance of mental illnesses: "The charge of the asylum was to bring discipline to the victims of disorganized society. To this end it had to isolate itself and its members from chaotic conditions" (Rothman 1971, p. 138). Additionally, asylums would provide the insane with a setting within which to recover from their illnesses: "Behind the asylum walls medical superintendents would create and administer a calm, steady, and rehabilitative routine" (Rothman 1971, p. 138). A highly ordered, predictable environment with a limited array of simple tasks and experiences would promote a reordering of the ill person's mind, paving the way for a successful return to society.

The idea that social conditions could give rise to insanity was a radical departure from the beliefs of colonial times. Viewed as an act of God, insanity required no other explanation in colonial society and was not regarded as accessible to human intervention. By contrast, early nineteenth century observers situated in rapidly growing urban centers believed that insanity was becoming more common and saw this rise in prevalence in conjunction with dramatic dislocations in the society as a whole. This is not to say that the medical community of the times thought of insanity only in its social aspect. Indeed, the prevailing belief was that careful investigation of the brain of deceased insane persons would yield evidence of damage to the tissue of the brain, except that the damage might be too subtle to detect with contemporary medical methods. However, those putative physical changes were thought of as the end result of societal stress and chaos on the human organism. Even those who allowed for the possibility of hereditary influences held societal contributions in a more primary position:

> Heredity, declared Samuel Woodward, "never results in alienation of mind without the intervention of exciting causes. If the exciting causes of the disease are avoided, the strongest predisposition need not result in insanity." (Rothman 1971, p. 126)

It was therefore to social forces that medical workers of the times directed their energies, on the premise that altering those forces would alter the risk of mental illness and perhaps its subsequent course. Again, note the determination of the medical workers and their lay collaborators to minister to the insane. If they pointed to social causes of mental illness, it was in the interest of healing. If anyone was blamed, it was the nation as a whole and then only to mobilize a reparative response among the citizenry.

Asylum Treatment and the Family

In this ideological climate, the family was looked on as an indirect, passive agent to the onset of mental illness. If the principal cause of insanity was the disarray of American society, the family was at fault for not having shielded the patient sufficiently:

> The family was the one institution that psychiatrists believed might have calmed the frantic spirit at loose in the community. A well-ordered family could protect its charge from the disordered society, inoculating the child against the disease before he suffered exposure. Instead, it brought the germs right into the cradle. Whether indulgent or neglectful or hypersensitive to success, the family failed to discipline its charges. (Rothman 1971, p. 121)

It is important to note that the family was not thought of as the germ, but rather as having allowed the germ to slip through. We see here a rather circumscribed criticism of the family. Others would have to shield those who fell ill because the family had proved insufficient to the task. Only much later would the family come to be seen as an offending agent in itself. In these earlier days, entry into the institution was seen as serving to protect the patient from the confusion and pressure of the wider society. Contact with that society outside the walls was discouraged as a part of the effort to invoke a quiet, orderly existence, and separation from relatives was but one element in that process. Rothman cited Isaac Ray on the importance of isolation:

> While at large, the patient is every moment exposed to circumstances
> that maintain the morbid activity of his mind [and] the dearer the
> friend, the greater the emotion. . . . In the hospital, on the other
> hand, he is beyond the reach of all these causes of excitement. (Rothman 1971, p. 137)

He goes on to cite Edward Jarvis in like manner:

> How else could the insane escape the cares and anxieties of business
> . . . the affairs of the town . . . the movements of religious, political
> and other associations. . . . Hospitals are the proper places for the in-
> sane . . . the cure and care of the insane belong to proper public in-
> stitutions. (Rothman 1971, p. 137)

Visits by family were limited as a part of the general policy of maintaining asylum for the patient until the illness abated. If the family had proved incapable of shielding the germ before the onset of the illness, they might unwittingly bring it in with them, as if on their clothes. Too much news of the world of politics or business, or of the advances or travails of compatriots or competitors, would intrude into that healing repose.

> Medical superintendents also discouraged the exchange of letters,
> fearing that news from home might intrude on the calm and regular
> routine of the asylum and upset the patient's stability . . . they were
> eager to preserve the insularity of their domain. "Long and tender
> letters," warned Ohio's superintendent William Awl, "containing
> some ill-timed news, or the melancholy tiding of sickness and death
> . . . may destroy weeks and months of favorable progress." (Rothman
> 1971, pp. 142–143)

Thus, families would be discouraged from having contact with the patient, save for short visits, until the patient was sufficiently improved to go home.

There is very little direct evidence as to the effects of these practices on the relationship between family and patient. Relatives had little access to the patient during the height of the illness; thus, it was impossible for the family to learn how to respond constructively to illness-related behavior. Because they were actively discouraging contact with any part of the patient's outside life that might "carry the germ," the doctors of the asylum era would not have regarded it as in any way worthwhile to listen to the family's observations during contacts with the inmate, let alone to make recommendations to the family as to how to conduct themselves during visits. The general reaction of the doctor, on hearing of an inmate's distress after a visit, was to discourage further visiting, at least until the illness had abated. The idea that some alteration in the family's conduct during the visit could lead to a more benevolent contact would not have been entertained. The idea that a visit might actually promote recovery was beyond thinking. And the idea that loss of contact was having any impact on relatives—that the inmate was missed or needed at home, that loved ones were grieving the loss of his or her contribution to the family—would have seemed altogether irrelevant to the mission of the asylum.

Throughout the period in which the asylums were gaining the ascendancy, families were learning how to participate in the new orientation. Relatives would do so in the sincere belief that they were bringing a loved one to the site of the best available medical care. As the whole society embraced the psychology of asylum, families learned to take note of the earliest manifestations of deviance or reappearance of deviance. Then, instead of tolerating that deviance, or talking the patient through it or engaging him or her in some calming activity, relatives would immediately seek medical attention. This pattern of response to the manifestations of mental illness could be learned as soon as an asylum was near at hand. It was also vigorously encouraged by the medical community of the times:

> The first postulate of the asylum program was the prompt removal of the insane from the community. As soon as the first symptom of the disease appeared, the patient had to enter a mental hospital. Medical superintendents unanimously and without qualification asserted the treatment within the family was doomed to fail. (Rothman 1971, p. 137)

What was lost with the advance of a policy of immediate removal was any skillfulness families had acquired in living day-to-day with their mentally ill relatives and through the various phases of the illness. In the era before asylums were available, and before removal came to be seen as a positive, restorative act, placement in an institution would have been viewed by families as a last, desperate response to extremes of social disruptiveness in the ill person's conduct. Instead of employing prompt removal, relatives and neighbors in those earlier times might well have drawn on an array of interpersonal coping skills designed to restore order without removal. The most flagrant of these, including procedures for dealing with the mentally ill as witches, public corporal punishment, and incarceration, have reached our attention, largely due to the emphasis given to them by the early advocates of asylum. But a range of more mundane relational skills may also have been available to families and communities during the colonial era.

Prompt removal of the patient brought prompt removal of the conditions under which a family and a community could acquire and maintain skills for living with a mentally ill person. Presumably, these skills were once passed from generation to generation. No longer regarded as relevant in an asylum-oriented culture, these skills may have disappeared inside of one generation's lifetime.

RISE OF PSYCHOANALYTIC THEORIES OF SYMPTOM FORMATION

It is sheer conjecture at what point in the development of psychodynamic theory the first application to an understanding of major mental illnesses took place. But the precise chronicling of that development is less at issue here than the recognition that at some point, medical opinion shifted. Instead of being concerned that relatives would bring the germs of society with them on a visit, the superintendents came to the view that the family, and mothers in particular, were the germs outright. It was not the poison of a chaotic society but the poison of a chaotic (or cold, rejecting, intrusive, confusing) mothering figure that was now seen as the first cause of insanity. The idea presumably came along with the growing emphasis on early mother-child interaction in modeling personality development. If personality could be so affected, and if dramatic, incapacitating neuroses could arise from pathogenic parent-child interaction, then, in the belief of the times, so could psychotic symptoms arise from family interactions. And if less severe illnesses derived from disruptions at the age of 5 or so, then the psychoses must, of course, arise from disruptions still earlier in life.

Unlike the superintendents of the 1850s, their counterparts in the 1950s did not automatically believe that the offending environmental influence eventuated in physical alterations in brain tissue. Indeed, the classic neuropathological investigations of the early twentieth century, although taking place with technologies advanced for the time, had not turned up very impressive evidence of brain pathologies in psychotic patients. Studies of twins in the 1930s produced some evidence supporting genetic theories of transmission, but epidemiological methods had not advanced to the point that clinicians of the time could regard the evidence as solid. In this intellectual climate, in a nation with a strong fundamental preference for environmental theories, developmental theories of the psychoses quickly gained the ascendancy.

This combination of technical and theoretical developments in psychiatry combined to produce the first strands of a novel orientation toward the family, an orientation that was at once more specific in its attribution of responsibility for the illness and more embracing in its sanction of interaction—supervised interaction—between family and patient. The new approach appeared in the psychiatric literature for the first time with Hadju-Gines' (1940) characterization of mothers of schizophrenic women as cold and sadistic, and again in 1948 with Fromm-Reichmann's now-famous description of these mothers as rejecting and "schizophrenogenic." Especially in the case of Fromm-Reichmann, the account is so much a passing comment, an aside in an unrelated discourse, that one has the impression that she is discussing an idea familiar to her readers rather than breaking new ground. Perhaps the construct mother-as-pathogen was already firmly rooted. Perhaps the only novel development in 1948 was the coining of a term as a shorthand for the idea. In short order, a whole new line of investigation was underway. By the mid-1950s, some of the brightest investigators and clinicians of the time were switching from reliance on strict asylum policies to observed encounters between family and patient.

It is important to note that, as with the development of the asylum hospitals, these new practices were founded on a determination to heal. The course of insanity had not been appreciably altered with 100 years of asylum. Many patients improved only to become ill again on return to the open society. Even if the germ was out there somewhere, psychiatry could not claim to have discovered it or to have altered the chaos of society so as to reduce its prevalence. But in the 1950s, it suddenly seemed possible to discover the germ, for instead of having to look into all aspects of society, the new theory suggested one could look instead simply at family life. In its time, this was an optimistic hypothesis. In the intellectual climate of the times, psychiatry reasoned that "we should be glad to discover a germ in the family, for it will be far easier to disinfect the family than to disinfect the entire social order." And whereas much of society wanted little to do with the insane, many families were eager to accept more frequent and more extensive visits in exchange for the relatively small intrusion of being closely observed by the new investigators.

Family Therapy and the Family

Thus was the telescope refocused. The caretakers of the insane abandoned the rule of retreat and became interested in the smallest nuances of interaction between patient and relative. In former days, the observation of upset after a family visit was evidence that societal pressures had leaked through the imposed isolation. Now that same upset was taken as confirmation that the family was making the patient crazy. Some even claimed that certain families made efforts to drive a patient crazy. The reversal in perspective also gave rise to a new form of treatment. Whereas the patient's upset had been taken as evidence of the need for more careful and more complete isolation, now it served as substantiation of the need for specific efforts to alter the course of family interaction. The new clinicians promoted gatherings of the entire family, including the patient, singling out interactions preceding the patient's upset that were taken to be producing the upset, in hope of showing the family how not to drive the patient crazy. This, of course, was the beginning of what came to be known as family therapy.

Just as the theory of the psychoses underwent a reversal in the first half of the twentieth century, so also the effects of mental illness on the family underwent a parallel reversal. Instead of feeling guilty about not having protected the ill person from external pathogens, the family had to contend with the guilt of having been the pathogen. Instead of losing sight of the patient for long stretches of time behind the walls of the institution, the family had to confront the patient's most disorganized behavior during visits to the hospital, during family therapy sessions, and during the patient's furloughs into the community.

TRENDS TOWARD CARE IN THE COMMUNITY

By an accident of fate, these developments in psychoanalytic and family interaction theory were emerging at the same time that neuroleptic drugs were becoming available. The first licenses for the investigational use of chlorpromazine (Thorazine and others) were given in 1953, and within 2 years it was in regular use in the asylum hospitals of America. Early observers noted that the drug had dramatic calming and ordering effects. Patients long since consigned to a life of asylum were now seen as candidates for early discharge. Stimulated by these observations, the interest in asylums, which had long since lost their appeal as places of healing, gave way to a new wave of interest in community-based treatment for the mentally ill. Once removed from their communities, the mentally ill of America were now to be removed from their asylums.

As always, the interest of the doctors was to heal. Over decades of asylum treatment, it had become apparent that removal from society did not regularly achieve the desired result, and that the institutions had their own ill effects on the mentally ill. By the 1950s, experienced observers were noting that asylum life had profoundly disruptive effects on social skills of the mentally ill and on their ties to family and to the wider community. The concern emerged that some of the most devastating manifestations of mental illness—the lack of feeling and motivation, which would later come to be called negative symptoms—might be manifestations of exposure to institutional life with its attendant loss of personal dignity, personal autonomy, and affectional ties. So when the mental health pioneers of the 1950s reversed course, it was largely to shield their patients from the effects of institutional life.

Now, however, families faced a new kind of burden. The asylum superintendents had had little concern for the burden of the illness on the rest of the family, but at least the asylum afforded the mentally ill a place to live and lifted the burden of daily care from their families. With the shift to community-based care, families and neighborhoods were distinctly unprepared to reabsorb the former inmates, even if they were no longer overtly symptomatic. For 100 years, generations had learned to see signs of illness and to effect prompt removal. Collectively, they had forgotten how to live with a mentally ill person. The skills had not been passed along. Between their preoccupation with the ill effects of the asylum existence and their optimism for the new drug treatments, the superintendents of the 1950s and 1960s failed to attend to the family's need to learn anew. The hospital staff called on families to assume care-giving tasks and responsibilities without determining what knowledge and skills they brought to the task, and without regard for the impact of this new role on the lives of other family members. At first this meant that people who had been taught to forget the patient, to surrender all hopes of a return to significant interaction with the patient, were told that they should resume care-giving activities and try to recapture the lost relationship. Then, with increasing frequency, families began to experience the reverse phenomenon: they were encouraged to take patients home after short stays, so as not to allow any appreciable distance to develop, lest the patient lose the social skills necessary for or lose interest in community life. In neither case have families received very much in the way of information, support, advice, or respect for their other lives, which are essential if the family is to avoid sinking under the weight of these new care-giving responsibilities.

The experience of one family moving along this path illustrates how relatives can feel whipsawed by the philosophical and programmatic changes taking place within the mental health professions:

A young woman hospitalized for 2 years in a classic asylum hospital improved to the point that she could return to the community. She and her parents were told that it would be inadvisable for her to return to the parental home, even though the parents had assumed that this would be the next move and they were eager to have her home. She was transferred to a local halfway house. Two years later, the staff of the halfway house, including a newly hired recently graduated social worker, informed the woman and her parents that she must leave the house and strongly recommended that the parents take her back into their home. The parents were disinclined to accept this recommendation, recalling that they had been cautioned against such a move by the hospital staff 2 years earlier. Reacting to the parents' reluctance as if they were rejecting their daughter, the halfway house staff stated that the parents had had enough of a reprieve and must now take their daughter home where, in the revised opinion, she belonged.

CONTEMPORARY TREATMENT PERSPECTIVES

Biological Orientation

If the trends toward family theories, family therapy, and community-based care have been burdensome to families, another development with more mixed effects has been the renaissance in the biological orientation toward severe mental illness. The news that conditions like the schizophrenias and the affective disorders have strong biochemical, genetic, or other psychobiological roots has largely been greeted with relief and optimism among families of the mentally ill. The evidence of biological roots of mental illness has allowed families to lift the yoke of blame, to cease shamefully hiding the patient and themselves, and to rebuild a position of respect and advocacy in their communities. But this same information has also constituted a betrayal of a kind for many relatives. Devoted families who endured waves of self-recrimination and criticism from professionals and who made massive sacrifices in an effort to purge the germ in their life have had to face the realization that all that careful self-scrutiny may have been for naught. The effect is equivalent to being released from prison after 10 years and told that you never committed the crime, that it was all a mistake.

Remnants of Formerly New Wave Treatments

Asylum. We are now several decades past the close of the era in which long-term asylum from presumed noxious forces in the environment was the prevailing philosophy of care for the mentally ill. Yet we are surrounded by concrete reminders of that era. Most of the places in which the mentally ill reside during the active phases of their illness are large and institutional in nature. Despite evidence coming from several demonstration projects showing that acutely ill patients can be cared for in smaller home-life environments, including in some cases the patient's own home, the vast majority of care during this phase still occurs in hospitals, organized on Jarvis' principle that "the cure and care of the insane belong to proper public institutions" (Rothman 1971, p. 137). In many, perhaps most, hospitals, social exchanges between the patient and his or her family and friends are curtailed by visiting rules that are more stringent than for the non-psychiatric parts of the same institutions. It is not unheard of even at this late date for families to be barred from visiting for some pro-scribed first part of the patient's stay. And it is even more common to observe hospital staff reacting to postvisit upset in the patient by limiting further visiting.

The situation in supportive aftercare is not substantially different. Many halfway houses and board-and-care homes assume an avoidant posture toward families and friends of residents. It is the unusual community setting that proactively embraces involvement of families in the life of the residence. Even though these settings are located in communities, they are rarely part of the community in any meaningful sense. In all respects, they function to the greatest extent possible in isolation from their surroundings.

Psychoanalytic theories.   Psychoanalytic ideas about the etiology of the psychoses are abundantly in evidence in clinical settings. Those of us involved in the National Alliance for the Mentally Ill (NAMI) who work in clinical facilities can bear witness to the regularity with which families of the chronically mentally ill are still being represented as pathogenic. Case conference descriptions of parents of young adult patients continue to be collections of unredeeming characterizations:

> Mother is a 60-year-old Anglo-Saxon Protestant with a high school diploma who retired from her clerical job in 1983 in order to care for the patient. Mother is a marginally reflective woman who believes in "the power of positive thinking," and sets goals for herself such as "being more assertive" and setting limits on her children's demands on her time. She is anxious and tangential and avoids family conflict by accommodating others. (Personal communication, New York Hospital, 1986)

A similar preoccupation with unfavorable aspects of the parents of the mentally ill is manifest even in less formal situations. The following passage is an account of a discussion transpiring among five psychiatrists who had met informally for 10 years as a peer support group of which I was a member:

> Through a series of referrals, three of the psychiatrists had had direct contact with a family that had two mentally ill young-adult children. On this particular occasion, Dr. C began discussing the

most recent referral, which led to a most surprising discovery. One of the sons, now having completed a long and successful course of individual psychotherapy with Dr. Q, indicated a desire to work out some unresolved issues with his parents. Dr. Q recommended he contact Dr. C, whom he described as a psychiatrist interested in family therapy. The son scheduled a session with his parents, unaware that his mother had been the first-grade teacher of Dr. C's two children. Dr. C discovered this when the mother called him before the first scheduled session, revealing that in speaking further to her son she had just realized that they knew each other. Arrangements were then made for a referral to another therapist. In the meeting with his colleagues, he described how shocked and saddened he was to learn of the personal tragedies in this woman's life, tragedies that were all the more poignant in view of her brilliance as a teacher. This woman, he recounted, had been the first to notice how very exceptional his own two children were. Her attention to their talents and her manifest devotion to them made her, in his view, an exceptional person. He was grateful for all she had done for his children. Dr. Q at this point remarked, "She's done a lot for her own children too: eight psychotic breaks!" He was ready to defend this view based on work with the son, until Dr. G intervened, challenging the use of such anamnestic material as was available to Dr. Q through the psychotherapy of the son as support for that statement. Dr. Q then immediately acceded.

Dr. Q was giving voice to a residual attitude that lives on in the formal and informal communications of many clinicians who are looking after mentally ill people. The attitude is less evident in the descriptions of actual psychotherapy of such patients than in communications about the family and specifically about the parents of the patient. Thus, this attitude does not seem to result from data that are integrated into the treatment plan, but rather exists as a dissociated or independent representation. As such, it has much in common with prejudice.

Family therapy is in no better position in this regard. At the opening session of the 1985 Annual Meeting of the American Association of Marriage and Family Therapists, Dr. Mara Selvini-Palazzoli (1985) addressed 2,000 family therapists on the topic "Toward a General Theory of Psychotic Family Games." In her address, she stated with conviction—really in the manner of a foregone conclusion—that one looks for "dirty family games" wherever one finds schizophrenia. One looks for such games because they must perforce exist, accounting for the illness in the patient. The attitude is apparent as well in the more careful family research literature. Rodnick et al. (1984) favored an interpersonal learning model for the interpretation of results from the UCLA Family Project, although one of the predictors they identified (communication deviance) can also be interpreted as a marker of attentional mechanisms not unlike the smooth-pursuit measure of Holzman et al. (1984) and the distractibility measures of Spring (1985). This preference is manifest in an interview published in the *New York Times* in which Goldstein discussed the preliminary findings of the UCLA Family Project:

> "The parents of these kids engaged in character assassinations," said Dr. Michael J. Goldstein, the director of the study. "Instead of criticizing what the child had done, they would make a personal attack, saying, 'You're no good,' which damages the child's self-esteem. The parents also were highly intrusive, telling the kid what he thinks or feels without regard to what the kid says, things like, 'You know, you really don't like that kid you go around with.' The kid can easily become unsure of what he really does think. These parents also spoke in a way that leaves the child feeling confused or uncertain. They'd use words inappropriately, or undercut what they'd said by denying it or making it ambiguous. The result is to leave the child feeling that he doesn't know what to believe, with a shaken sense of reality. Further, the child learns a peculiar style of reasoning, and a chaotic way of thinking." (Goleman 1984)

During informal conversations on two occasions within the last year, two major figures within the family field (one in Washington, one in New York) have confided to me that "we do the same things we've always done: we just don't talk about it the same way." All the developments regarding the positive role of the family notwithstanding, these two individuals persevere in privately held derogatory orientations toward families.

As illustrated by the following incident, the same attitude also persists among informed lay people:

> Recently I was consulted by a woman whose son was ill with cancer. One day, in the course of scheduling appointments, I had occasion to reveal that I would soon be giving a paper. When she asked about the topic, I indicated that the paper would focus on the experience of families of the mentally ill. Comparing the predicament of such families with her own, she remarked, "Now those parents have, I think, the most difficult problem imaginable, because they have caused the problem themselves!"

This cultured, intelligent woman spoke sorrowfully and with complete conviction on the matter, giving voice to the prevailing belief among the citizenry. One even sees this attitude among families of the mentally ill on occasion, and it becomes necessary to challenge a parent's wish to have been at fault:

> When faced with an adult child's psychosis, some parents seem to reason that "if I made it happen, I can make it go away." The poignancy of this magical line of thinking was revealed to me by one mother who tearfully remarked, "I was even willing to be wrong if it would make Christine better." (Terkelsen 1982)

Some parents will spontaneously report a range of disagreeable interactions with the patient, believing, with their counterparts in the citizenry, that they caused the illness.

Perhaps professionals who give voice to these ideas are speaking
more from basic societal assumptions than from science. Whatever
the explanation, it is a fiction to think that the mental health professions have recovered or can easily recover from their attachment to
pejorative attitudes toward families of the mentally ill. The ideas are
very powerful and very attractive. They are alive and well everywhere
in America.

Deinstitutionalization. As for remnants of deinstitutionalization,
one has only to listen to the discussions in support groups of local
NAMI chapters to hear how frequently families are confronted with
premature discharges from hospitals. Families have begun to realize
that they do not have to accept the decision of the hospital staff when
they believe the patient is not ready to return home. Nor must they
accept the hospital's decision to send their loved one to live in some
ramshackle single-room-occupancy hotel. Families now know that such
steps are often in violation of state law or the standards of practice
set out by the Joint Commission on the Accreditation of Hospitals,
with which hospitals must comply. But families have had to familiarize
themselves with the law in this domain precisely because many hospitals have continued to pressure them to accept a patient into their
home for purposes of avoiding prolonged institutional exposure.

Families also continue to encounter pressure at the other end of
hospital care as well. In many communities, crisis teams have been
established, not so much to respond to emerging trouble in the community as to divert patients from inpatient care. For this reason, the
teams get low ratings in many communities on responsiveness to situations perceived as emergencies by families. Once it becomes apparent that the family wants the patient placed in a hospital, the team
becomes unresponsive.

A derivative form of resistance to admission is now emerging as
local mental health planners become aware of the preliminary results
of the psychoeducational programs of Falloon et al. (1984) and Anderson et al. (1986). Increasing numbers of public agencies are offering
educational programs to families, not as a service of informational
value, but in the belief that it is an intervention that will diminish the
rate of readmission to the hospital. The program becomes a contemporary representation of the deinstitutionalization movement.

OPTIMAL RELATIONS BETWEEN FAMILIES
AND PROVIDERS

What is striking about the current array of settings, both hospital and community-based programs, is the extent to which the clinical staff think and live and plan for patients as if they constituted a virtual replacement for the patient's family. Some readers will immediately think of exceptions to this general observation, but it is worth noting the prevailing mental set of those working within the settings that constitute the professional side of contemporary care giving. These settings do not possess policy and program features that seek to involve the patient's natural support system in a collaborative interaction. For example, not until its 10th year of operation did the major community residence provider in Westchester County, New York, invite families to attend a meeting to discuss the philosophy and practices of the organization. Inviting the family in for family therapy or multiple family therapy sessions or even for family night or psycho-educational workshops is a far cry from the kind of collaboration I am talking about. As valuable as these experiences can be for families in learning about illness and about the day-to-day problems and limitations of a mentally ill person, they do not approach the kind of joint work that would constitute the end of the psychology of asylum in the vast majority of contemporary care settings.

I do not mean to condemn asylum per se. Some patients are so sensitive to the complexity and emotional intensity of ordinary community life or so lacking in basic social skills, either at some point in their illness or for the entire duration of the illness, as to require settings that provide asylum in the true sense of being apart from the community as a whole (Lamb 1979, 1981; Bachrach 1985). Other patients living in settings that provide and encourage ready access to family and community life will episodically disengage from those involvements, usually in an effort to self-regulate the extent of complexity and emotional intensity to which they expose themselves. There is a need for families and clinicians to evolve a culture of collaboration, a habit of including each other in their thoughts and their actions on behalf of the patient. Day-to-day life with a mentally ill person varies across a wide spectrum of complexity. Some families manage this life with conventional psychiatric services that offer only peripheral involvement of clinicians. Others can take it on with daily involvement of clinicians. For many others, the impact on other family members is too large to be tolerated, and the family cannot care for its ill member at home. Too often, decisions about what is good for a patient are made without direct involvement of the family. The disinclination to involve families in decision making may have gone unnoticed in the era when families were told to forget the patient; now, however, decisions made by clinicians are likely to have an impact directly and immediately on some aspect of the family's life. Families should be invited to participate in treatment planning sessions on a status equal to that of any professional community agency that is involved with the patient. As one example of this kind of collaboration, Altman (1983) described the use of a joint conference at or near the point of discharge in which inpatient staff convene together with family, patient, and representatives of every agency that will have some part in the aftercare plan. Called *collaborative discharge planning*, the method showed promise in reducing early returns to the hospital in a chronic population. The event places key relatives and agency staff on an equal footing as they begin or resume their various care-giving tasks vis-à-vis the patient.

If we are to maintain the spirit of the trend toward community care, the vast majority of programs and facilities should now be fostering regular engagement of patient and family, staff, and neighbors in activities that are elements of ordinary day-to-day community life. I am referring to activities that fulfill maintenance functions or situations in which patients together with others in the natural and illness-related support systems are engaged in learning to perform such maintenance functions collaboratively.

My views on this matter derive from at least 15 years of daily contact with mentally ill persons living in community settings, which has left me with the conviction that, at any point in time, most are capable of engaging in numerous activities that characterize the citizenry. Further, they can do so in conjunction with the citizenry provided they have access to a linking person within the citizenry—someone with whom they can easily assume the status of an ill or impaired person, to whom they can reveal the exhaustion, the terror, and the despair that emerge in the course of attempts to function as part-time citizens.

The great disadvantage of asylum, in this regard, is the dissociation of the two realities frequented by the mentally ill person. First the patient is asked to live in the universe of illness, with other ill persons and with health professionals and their delegates. Then the patient is encouraged to enter the universe of wellness and to move around among the citizenry. Much has been made of the observation that severely mentally ill persons do not generalize learnings from one environment to another very well. This observation is cited as the explanation of the difficult transit faced by the mentally ill on leaving institutions to live in community-based settings. Presumably, failure to generalize has its roots in the impairment in object constancy, that is, in the inability or limited ability to maintain a clear and durable internal image of oneself—one's identity, one's status in relation to others, and the differential interactional requirements of various social situations—in the face of variable and often discontinuous environmental signals and demands. Something about mental illness, to a greater extent than other illnesses, makes it demanding to the extreme for the ill person to wear two or more hats.

If failure to generalize is a valid explanation of the failures in transit from hospital to community, it is also valid in understanding the difficulties of those now living in the community and facing daily transit from settings in which they have the status and identity of *patienthood*, to those in which they are regarded as *citizens*. The latter transit is just as demanding, perhaps even more demanding than the former. It is for this reason that careful attention must be given to the construction of daily, ordinary linkages—concretely in evidence to the patient in the form of visible, mutually respectful interactions—between family, program staff, and neighbors, i.e., representatives of all the types of social statuses that the patient assumes in the course of traveling through a day's ordinary encounters. This requirement, of course, points to certain types of training experiences, for professionals and for families, that are not generally available at present. In part, it is our task to characterize what those training experiences should be and who must make them available and in what settings.

REFERENCES

Altman H: A collaborative approach to discharge planning for chronic mental patients. Hosp Community Psychiatry 34:641–642, 1983

Anderson CM, Reiss DJ, Hogarty GE: Schizophrenia and the Family. New York, Guilford, 1986

Bachrach LL: Asylum and chronically ill psychiatric patients. Am J Psychiatry 141:975–978, 1985

Falloon IRH, Boyd JL, McGill CW: Family Care of Schizophrenia. New York, Guilford, 1984

Fromm-Reichmann F: Notes on the development of treatment of schizophrenics by psychoanalytic psychotherapy. Psychiatry 11:263–273, 1948

Goleman D: Schizophrenia: early signs found. New York Times, December 11, 1984

Hadju-Gines L: Contributions to the etiology of schizophrenia. Psychoanal Q 27:421–428, 1940

Holzman PH, Solomon CM, Levin S, et al: Pursuit eye movement dysfunction in schizophrenia: family evidence for specificity. Arch Gen Psychiatry 41:136–139, 1984

Lamb HR: The new asylum in the community. Arch Gen Psychiatry 36:129–134, 1979

Lamb HR: Maximizing the Potential of Board and Care Homes (New Directions for Mental Health Services: Issues in Community Residential Care, No 11). Edited by Budson RD. San Francisco, CA, Jossey-Bass, 1981

Rodnick EH, Goldstein MJ, Lewis JM, et al: Parental communication style, affect, and role as precursors of offspring schizophrenia—spectrum disorders, in Children at Risk for Schizophrenia: A Longitudinal Perspective. Edited by Watt NF, Anthony EJ, Wynne LC, et al. Cambridge, Cambridge University Press, 1984

Rothman DJ: The Discovery of the Asylum: Social Order and Disorder in the New Republic. Boston, Little, Brown, 1971

Selvini-Palazzoli M: Toward a general model of psychotic family games. Paper presented at the annual meeting of the American Association of Marriage and Family Therapists, New York, October 17, 1985

Spring B: Distractibility in schizophrenics and relatives. Paper presented in New Research at the annual meeting of the American Psychiatric Association, Dallas, TX, May 21, 1985

Terkelsen KG: The straight approach to a knotty problem: managing parental guilt about psychosis, in Questions and Answers in the Practice of Family Therapy, Vol 2. Edited by Gurman AS. New York, Brunner/Mazel, 1982 pp 179–183

Continuing Problems Between Mental Health Professionals and Families of the Mentally Ill

H. Richard Lamb, M.D.

Dr. Terkelsen has very thoughtfully and eloquently described the processes that have led to the tensions that exist between families of schizophrenic patients and mental health professionals and the heavy emotional costs of these tensions to families.

I agree that families are still being blamed, though perhaps more subtly, for their relatives' illnesses. On the current scene, expressed emotion (EE) serves as an excellent example. A detailed critique of EE research can be found elsewhere (Kanter et al. 1987), and I will confine myself here to some brief remarks without giving all of the evidence. In short, however, nowhere is there evidence that the "expressed emotion of families" causes relapse in schizophrenic patients. Despite this, the EE construct has been used implicitly, and sometimes explicitly, to blame families for exacerbations of schizophrenia.

DOES EE CAUSE RELAPSE?

Almost since the inception of EE research, there has been controversy about whether the EE variable reflects the family's effect on the patient or the patient's effect on the family. Leff and Vaughn (1985) have asserted that relatives' emotional attitudes have been firmly established as a causal factor in schizophrenic relapse." They offer "conclusive evidence" that EE's impact on outcome is independent of patient variables. Many mental health professionals have uncritically accepted their interpretation of the EE data and believe that EE reflects a stressful family situation that precipitates acute psychotic relapse and interferes with rehabilitative efforts.

Suggesting that EE is instead a family reaction to patient behavior, Vaughn and Leff (1976) earlier reported that 62% of the patients in their study and 75% of the patients in the study by Brown et al. (1972) either displayed behavior disturbing to family members (in the 3 months before admission) and lived with high-EE families or did not exhibit disturbing behavior and lived with low-EE families. More recent studies have examined more closely the EE construct and brought into question the more simplistic cause-and-effect speculation. For instance, Miklowitz et al. (1983) studied patient characteristics as well as measures of EE in relatives. High global levels of EE were not associated with premorbid psychosocial functioning or levels of residual symptomatology after discharge. These investigators obtained significant results only when they separately examined the dimensions of criticism and overinvolvement. They found that patients from "emotionally overinvolved" families manifested two characteristics suggestive of poor prognosis: poor premorbid psychosocial functioning and a greater level of residual symptomatology after discharge. They speculated that "overinvolvement" may represent an accommodation to the presence of a child with a long history of social dysfunction.

Looking separately at patients with families displaying critical attitudes, Miklowitz et al. (1983) found that these patients manifested comparatively higher levels of premorbid adjustment and less residual symptomatology, suggesting that these patients have more favorable prognoses. They speculated that critical parental behaviors may reflect a tendency for parents to react with anger and disappointment to patients of whom more was expected. These findings suggest that high levels of the EE component attitudes may be largely an appropriate, or at least expectable, reaction of relatives to extremely difficult situations and behaviors.

Nevertheless, the popular professional usage of high EE implies a family that is critical, hostile, and overinvolved. This association is explicitly encouraged by Leff et al. (1982), who argued that although clinicians cannot obtain the "long and arduous" training needed to reliably rate EE, they can readily identify high-EE families even without a familiarity with the concepts of criticism and overinvolvement. They go on to outline archetypes of both high- and low-EE families on the basis of their clinical experience. Briefly, low-EE families are empathic, patient, calm, and respectful, whereas high-EE familes are intrusive, critical, excitable, and overprotective. In their view, the former group is helpful to schizophrenic patients, whereas the latter group is harmful. Along these lines, in their recent book, Leff and Vaughn (1985) concluded their discussion with five case vignettes of extremely overinvolved families that in their view illustrate their argument that EE may be an etiological factor in schizophrenia. It is not surprising, then, that families feel blamed by professionals using the EE construct.

With regard to treatment strategies based on the EE construct, some investigators have made their specific focus that of lowering EE levels. However, family intervention strategies by other teams of investigators that offer relatives education, support, and advice without focusing on lowering EE levels have demonstrated beneficial results (Goldstein 1981; Falloon and Pederson 1985). Thus, there is little evidence that lowering EE, apart from the general education and professional support offered by all psychoeducational modalities, is the specific therapeutic ingredient influencing patient outcome.

I believe that treatment strategies based on the EE construct tend to (implicitly or explicitly) blame relatives for the level of family tensions. Such approaches may also suggest to patients they are not capable of controlling their behavior and do not encourage them to develop more socially acceptable behaviors and life-styles.

PUTTING FAMILIES INTO PERSPECTIVE— FOR PATIENTS AND PROFESSIONALS

In recent years, some authors have focused on the extent to which denial and distortion interfere with the patient's perception of his or her interpersonal environment. This issue has been relatively neglected in family research (Heinrichs and Carpenter 1983). Pursuing a similar train of thought, Arieti (1974) observed that schizophrenic patients tend to attribute to their parents full responsibility for their illness and their despair, absolving themselves from guilt and closing off examination of their own part in the development of illness. Unfortunately, many mental health professionals have accepted these perceptions of the family in toto as accurate accounts of historical events. Arieti (1975) believes that generally the patient's view is highly distorted and exaggerated; it is the therapist's job to help patients get their parents into perspective and stop blaming others for all their troubles. Patients need to recognize the role of others in their lives, but they also need to assume some responsibility for what happened to them in the past and especially for their current and future actions.

It is equally important for professionals to get families into perspective. Families should be seen as persons who have valuable ideas and knowledge. Many mental health professionals give lip service to the importance of families and their organizations. However, in clinical situations this attitude often does not seem to have filtered down to the actual work with schizophrenic patients. Clinicians often discount families' histories of patients' illnesses and what approaches and treatments have worked in the past.

Impact of Unrealistic Expectations

Unrealistic expectations of professionals have created additional burdens for both patients and families. The fact that the chronically mentally ill have been deinstitutionalized does not mean they no longer need social support, and protection and relief, either periodic or continuous, from the pressures of life. In short, most need varying degrees of asylum and sanctuary *in the community* (Lamb and Peele 1984). Unfortunately, because the old state hospitals were called asylums, the word asylum took on a bad, almost sinister, connotation. Only in recent years has the word again become a respectable part of our language with which one can denote the function of providing asylum, rather than asylum as a place.

The concept of asylum and sanctuary becomes important because, although some chronically mentally ill patients eventually attain high levels of social and vocational functioning, many others cannot meet simple demands of living on their own, even with long-term rehabilitative help. Many consciously limit their exposure to external stimuli and pressure, not from laziness but from a well-founded fear of failure. Professionals must realize that whatever degree of rehabilitation is possible for each patient cannot take place unless support and protection—whether in the form of family, treatment program, therapist, or board-and-care home—are provided at the same time. If this need for asylum and sanctuary in the community is not taken into account, living in the community at all may not be possible for many patients, and families and patients will experience an unnecessary and inappropriate sense of failure.

More Assertiveness Needed

I agree that professionals have much to learn from families and about families. But it is, in my opinion, a problem that requires more than simply further education of professionals. Professionals do not give up very easily their cherished beliefs, their priorities, and their power.

Dr. Terkelsen has pointed out that in spite of all the verbiage, the psychogenic theories of the etiology of schizophrenia and, more recently, similar theories that speak not so much to cause but rather to what precipitates acute exacerbations of schizophrenia are still widely held. And families still get the blame. The example of EE has, I believe, demonstrated that. Moreover, schizophrenia is still not the highest priority in public mental health; with many mental health professionals it is not even high on their list. And remaining "in charge" of both public policy and individual treatment without interference from families is still a power issue commonly found among mental health professionals.

Educating professionals and cultivating their good will are commendable and helpful, but grossly insufficient if research in and treatment of schizophrenia are to be truly elevated to their rightful place in mental health. Parents' organizations that got off to an auspicious start (Lamb and Oliphant 1978) have begun to falter. They have not maintained a degree of assertiveness sufficient for the task at hand. Even worse, they have at times allowed themselves to be co-opted and manipulated (Lamb et al. 1986).

Acceptance at Last

Parents have felt disliked and disapproved of for so long that there is a tendency for many, when shown some kindness and respect, to lose their perspective and become distracted from their main goals of improving treatment and services for the chronically mentally ill. Thus, parents have been put on boards of directors of organizations dealing with mental health and on mental health advisory boards, have been asked to contribute chapters in books, and have been invited to speak at professional meetings. At last they feel some acceptance. This is all the more important because they often felt very isolated from people generally for a long time (as happens when one has a mentally ill child). Under these circumstances, it is understandable that many parents will lose sight of the fact that some of the very persons and organizations that are embracing them are those who have been and continue to be obstacles to the provision of adequate and appropriate services to their schizophrenic relatives. In the glow of this seeming acceptance, the militancy of families frequently subsides, and they become less aware of when they are being manipulated.

Families must be single-minded in their advocacy for having the needs of schizophrenic patients met. They should learn from the example of the parents of the developmentally disabled, who are militant and unswerving (and very successful) in their efforts to improve the lot of the developmentally disabled. Parents of schizophrenic patients are often persuaded that they should champion other causes both in and out of mental health: "You must not be selfish by focusing only on schizophrenics." Not so the parents of the developmentally disabled. They advocate and work almost exclusively for "their own" and cannot be dissuaded from this course. The result has been a proliferation of services and increased funding for the developmentally disabled.

Now that families of schizophrenic patients have gained some recognition and acceptance, many say, "We do not want to be adversaries to the system. We want them to like us. You catch more flies with honey than with vinegar." Not so the families of the developmentally disabled. They may at times use honey, but those who stand in their way usually experience the force of their determination and dedication.

Families in the glow of their new "status" in the mental health establishment must not forget that a sizable proportion of mental health professionals have little interest in treating the chronically mentally ill and experience the treatment of schizophrenia as an unrewarding, frustrating experience that offers little hope for a positive outcome (Mirabi et al. 1985). Instead, many of these professionals may want to use public mental health funds to treat the healthy but unhappy, to do "insight" therapy with neurotic patients and those with character disorders, to attempt to combat poverty and to cure other ills of society, and to focus on the problems in the schools. Families of schizophrenic patients, on the other hand, are the champions of the chronically mentally ill and are the leading advocates for the treatment of chronic schizophrenia being the first and foremost priority of public mental health. Thus, these families are an obstacle to funding for causes favored by many health professionals. Mental health professionals may accept families as partners in these causes; then these families often begin to feel that they are being narrow and selfish if they insist that services for schizophrenic persons be the primary task for public mental health.

Families have gained a vast amount of insight through their support organizations. Families have gained knowledge from attending conferences. Families have not, however, in many ways made much progress in dealing with professionals. The highest priority of families of schizophrenic patients is to be listened to by society and by professionals, and to have a significant impact in terms of changes in the system.

WHAT DOES THE FUTURE HOLD?

Is the family movement in jeopardy of losing its effectiveness? It seems to me that it is, and that the following questions need to be posed. Can families be more assertive and single-minded in their advocacy for their schizophrenic relatives even if it means experiencing less of the "acceptance" from professionals and others that they have yearned for for so long? Can they rely less on the good will of professionals and more on their own potential political power? Can they maintain their own separate identities and not let themselves be co-opted by groups, such as professionals and ex-patients, with other agendas? Can they say who they are? For instance, can they use the word schizophrenia when referring to their organization and their concerns? On the answers to these questions depends the future of the family self-help movement, and the prospects for effective advocacy for the chronically mentally ill. Who can and will fulfill this role of assertive advocacy if not the families of schizophrenic patients and their organizations?

REFERENCES

Arieti S: Interpretation of Schizophrenia. New York, Basic Books, 1974

Arieti S: Psychiatric controversy: man's ethical dimension. Am J Psychiatry 132:39–42, 1975

Brown GW, Birley JLT, Wing JK: Influence of family life on the course of schizophrenic disorders: a replication. Br J Psychiatry 121:241–258, 1972

Falloon IRH, Pederson J: Family management in the prevention of morbidity of schizophrenia—the adjustment of the family unit. Br J Psychiatry 147:156–163, 1985

Goldstein MJ (ed): New Developments in Interventions With Families of Schizophrenics (New Directions for Mental Health Services, No 12). San Francisco, CA, Jossey-Bass, 1981

Heinrichs DW, Carpenter WT: The coordination of family therapy with other treatment modalities for schizophrenia, in Family Therapy in Schizophrenia. Edited by McFarlane WR. New York, Guilford, 1983, pp 267–287

Kanter J, Lamb HR, Loeper C: Expressed emotion in families: a critical review. Hosp Community Psychiatry 38:374–380, 1987

Lamb HR, Oliphant E: Schizophrenia through the eyes of families. Hosp Community Psychiatry 29:803–806, 1978

Lamb HR, Peele R: The need for continuing asylum and sanctuary. Hosp Community Psychiatry 35:798–802, 1984

Lamb HR, Hoffman A, Hoffman F, et al: Families of schizophrenics: a movement in jeopardy. Hosp Community Psychiatry 37:353–357, 1986

Leff J, Vaughn C: Expressed Emotion in Families: Its Significance for Mental Illness. New York, Guilford, 1985

Leff JP, Kuipers L, Berkowitz R, et al: A controlled trial of social intervention in the families of schizophrenic patients. Br J Psychiatry 141:121–134, 1982

Miklowitz DJ, Goldstein MJ, Falloon IRH: Premorbid and symptomatic characteristics of schizophrenics from families with high and low levels of expressed emotion. J Abnorm Psychol 92:359–367, 1983

Mirabi M, Weinman ML, Magnetti SM, et al: Professional attitudes toward the chronically mentally ill. Hosp Community Psychiatry 36:404–405, 1985

Vaughn CE, Leff JP: The influence of family and social factors on the course of psychiatric illness: a comparison of schizophrenic and depressed neurotic patients. Br J Psychiatry 129:125–137, 1976

Chapter 2

The Family's Experience of Living With Mental Illness

Dale L. Johnson, Ph.D.

Families continue to be the primary caretakers of the mentally ill, and by all accounts, this is true not only in the United States but in other parts of the world. Estimates of the number of mentally ill persons who live with families vary from around 50% (Lamb and Oliphant 1978) to 73% (Goldman 1982). Most estimates fall into the 60–70% range (Arey and Warheit 1980; Minkoff 1978; Reynolds and Hoult 1984; Thompson and Doll 1982). Where it is a matter of policy that mentally ill persons released from hospitals return to families, the rates are even higher; for example, Hoenig (1974) reported that 87% of former patients were living with family members in his study of hospital and community programs in one English community.

These estimates are often based on the number of patients who return to families after leaving a hospital and do not, therefore, include those mentally ill persons who, although disturbed, have not been hospitalized. The estimates also do not give an adequate picture of the amount of involvement families have with their mentally ill relative even though the mentally ill person may not be living in the family home. This includes families who are in regular contact with persons who are hospitalized or living in alternative residences of one kind or another in the community. The estimates also do not include a proportion of the "homeless mentally ill" who are being sought by family members. From the standpoint of the family, many of the individuals in this last group have disappeared and may or may not return (Hatfield et al. 1984; Johnson 1985).

Families also lead the way in making decisions that treatment is necessary and locating suitable treatment facilities. Furthermore, al-

31

though not widely acknowledged by mental health professionals, it is often the family that must monitor the course of treatment in order to maintain quality and provide continuity of care.

HISTORICAL CHANGES IN VIEWS OF FAMILIES OF THE MENTALLY ILL

Within a rather short time, the views that professionals have held about the families of the mentally ill have changed radically. There appear to be three different perspectives, and each has been salient at a different time.

Attitudes and stigma. Research on families of the mentally ill in the 1950s and 1960s tended to emphasize attitudes toward the mentally ill. To some extent, this was part of a search for predictors of relapse and attempts to improve patient length of stay in the community. It was believed that family intolerance of mental illness might be related to relapse. The work of this era has been reviewed by Kreisman and Joy (1974) and by Rabkin (1974).

Etiology. In the absence of persuasive genetic, anatomical, physiological, or biochemical evidence for the etiology of the major mental disorders, psychological theories flourished. Freud, of course, set the stage with his theory of the origin of the neuroses in early childhood experience. He was guarded about the applicability of the theory for the major psychoses, but his followers have had no hesitation in assigning primary causality to the persons in the child's early environment, chiefly the mother. Fromm-Reichmann (1948) captured the essence of this way of thinking with her concept of the "schizophrenogenic mother" and provided the impetus for an entire course of research.

The work of Bateson et al. (1956) on the double bind and of Lidz and Lidz (1949) and Wynne and Singer (1963) on communication deviance introduced the "systems" approach to the mental sciences and spawned a new line of research on the families of the mentally ill as agents in the etiology of the illness.

Family members as persons. Apparently, the first consideration of the families of the mentally ill as possibly burdened, that is, as affected by living with the mentally ill person, was by Mandelbrote and Folkard (1961) in their study of deinstitutionalization in Sweden. This was followed by numerous studies in the United Kingdom also having to do with the impact on the family of reliance on community treatment of the mentally ill (Brown et al. 1966). This work eventually led to a formulation of the family as being involved, not as an etiological agent as it was assumed that the primary etiology was biochemical and/or genetic, but as an important factor in managing the environment of the mentally ill person. This, in turn, led to the development of training programs for families of the mentally ill, which were shown to be effective in reducing relapse rates (Vaughn and Leff 1976). This work has been replicated, with some modifications, in the United States (Anderson et al. 1986; Falloon et al. 1984).

At about the same time, the family advocacy movement was organized in 1979 into the National Alliance for the Mentally Ill (NAMI). Members of this organization have taken a strong stand in rejecting the family-environment etiological theories and have viewed family members as people who are heavily burdened by the care of a person or persons who suffer from a brain disorder and whose behavior is demanding, troublesome, and baffling.

I review in this chapter the literature that has accumulated during the third historical era having to do with family members' experience with mental illness. Several questions are raised, and the literature is examined for answers: What is there about mental illness that families find burdensome? What are the effects of living with mental illness on family members? What are the economic costs of mental illness? Under what conditions is the burden of mental illness high or low? In what way have mental health professionals had an impact on the burden of mental illness?

EXPERIENTIAL REALITIES OF LIVING WITH MENTAL ILLNESS

The term *mental illness* in this review will be used to include schizophrenia, major affective disorder, bipolar affective disorder, and borderline disorders. It does not include the various organic disorders or disorders of childhood.

The behaviors of mental illness are extremely variable from one mentally ill person to another and even for one person from time to time. The major features typically include delusions, hallucinations, thought disorder, lack of emotional feeling, listlessness, and apathy. There may be great affective changes, from despair to joy. Activity may vary from immobility to manic fervor. Judgment is often impaired and insight lacking. Violence to self or others is a possibility. Social judgment is impaired, leading to embarrassment to self and family members.

Because family members have a life history perspective on the disorder, their experience may be one of shock as the normal person becomes distinctly abnormal; or they may have seen the gradual deterioration of a person in the family who from birth seemed different and always needed help. The perspective across time also reveals that mental illness too often does not go away—the person may have well periods, but recurrence of the psychotic behaviors is common. Mental illness is often episodic, and very often chronic.

Families faced with mental illness for the first time are baffled and may be slow in coming to a decision for the need for professional help (Lefley 1987a). There is often a question of what is truly abnormal and what is normal deviance in adolescence or early adulthood, or merely deviance from family norms. The illness is enigmatic to family members and to mental health professionals, many of whom are reluctant to make a diagnosis until the disorder has been apparent for some time, leaving the family in a state of ambiguity. This ambiguity is in itself a source of stress.

Another characteristic of mental illness is that the person afflicted is typically quite unable to carry out conventional roles, such as those of wage earner, student, or homemaker, and is dependent on others. This dependence too is a source of conflict between the dependent person and the caretakers.

Sources of Information

The sources of information for this review of the impact of mental illness on family members are primarily from published surveys of two types: 1) surveys of persons who are members of NAMI or similar advocacy/self-help groups and 2) surveys of family members of clients of mental health service providers. The respondents to these two types of surveys differ in important ways, as do the clients who are the focus of attention. Surveys of NAMI members are highly similar in that the respondents tend to be women (70–80%), aged 50–70, well educated, of managerial or professional socioeconomic status, and married, widowed, or divorced. They report on sons (70–90%) who have typically had some college, but little employment, and who are unmarried. The other surveys usually do not report the sex of the respondent, but the sex distribution of the mentally ill family members is about equal, and they present a broad socioeconomic range. Because the NAMI member surveys have so often shown a preponderance of male mentally ill persons, some individuals have suggested that the major mental illnesses are more prevalent among males. A number of well-designed surveys of the population in general have found little evidence that this is true; males and females are approximately equally represented (Myers et al. 1984).

The differences in respondents and mentally ill persons found for the two types of surveys will require that surveys of family burden take these differences into consideration. It is possible that they will yield different results.

Effects on the Family in General

Most of the studies of the impact of mental illness on families do not make a distinction as to relationship. Presumably, a large number of these unspecified family members are parents, but spouses, siblings, children, and other relatives are included.

Objective burden. Numerous investigators have used the term *objective burden* to describe the patient behaviors that concern them most, that is, what they are worried about or what they perceive as abnormal. Surveys of NAMI members reveal a considerable variety of behaviors that are burdensome. Hatfield (1978) reported that her sample of 89 family members judged the following behaviors disturbing, in rank order: lacks motivation, handles money poorly, shows poor grooming and personal care, has unusual eating and sleeping habits, forgets to do things, talks without making sense, argues too much, refuses to take medication, thinks people talk about him or her, hears voices, and breaks and damages things. Spaniol et al. (1984) found in their sample (*n* = 140) that concern was greatest, in rank order, for schizophrenic symptoms, depression, listlessness and low energy, and aggressiveness. Creer and Wing (1975) conducted a similar survey in the United Kingdom. They found that the following behaviors were most frequently cited: social withdrawal, underactivity, lack of conversation, overactivity, few leisure interests, odd ideas, odd behavior, depression, neglect of appearance, and odd postures and movements. Lefley's (1987b) sample of 84 mental health professionals who had mentally ill relatives ranked as very important mood swings, disruption of household routines, social isolation, lack of motivation, poor handling of money, unusual sleep patterns, verbal abuse of others, and refusal to take medication.

Family members of patients receiving psychiatric treatment have also been the subjects of research on objective burden. Grad and Sainsbury (1968) received 319 completed questionnaires from family members in a study carried out in the United Kingdom. In rank order, they were concerned about uncooperative and contrary behaviors, restlessness, hypochondriacal preoccupations, odd or unreasonable behaviors, night disturbances, suicidal behaviors, violence, and unpleasant or objectionable speech or behaviors. Hoenig and Hamilton (1969), also working in the United Kingdom, reported that family members in their research found the following behaviors most burdensome: disturbing behavior, odd speech or ideas, apparent willful uncooperativeness, dangerousness to self or others, restlessness or talkativeness, unresponsiveness, and night wandering.

In a study of 125 family members of patients from three Ohio psychiatric hospitals, Thompson and Doll (1982) found the overall level of objective burden to be high. The most frequently mentioned components of this burden were that the disturbed family member required much supervision, was a financial burden, presented role strains, disrupted daily routines, and presented problems with neighbors. Smith (1969) also found a high level of burden among the families of mentally ill patients in Canada. The families in his study were most commonly concerned about behavior that was odd, required close supervision, and interfered with social or leisure activities. Objective burden was also assessed by Herz et al. (1976) in their study of 153 family members of patients hospitalized or living at home. The most commonly cited burdensome behaviors were that the patient contributed less money to the household than before the psychosis, the family had to assume additional responsibilities, much time was required to supervise the patient, and irritability or anger. In another study of families of patients in treatment, Fenton et al. (1979) found that patient behavior disrupted family activities, forced other family members to assume the patient's responsibilities, bothered others, and created financial problems.

Most of the patients in the above studies were schizophrenic. Schulz et al. (1982) investigated the impact of borderline and schizotypal personality disorders on families. The level of objective burden was high, with 80% of the families reporting moderate to severe burden. They were most troubled by patient anger and antisocial behaviors.

It is obvious from these surveys that the level of objective burden for families is high. This is true whether the respondents are members of advocacy groups such as NAMI or are the families of patients currently in treatment. The findings seem similar across nations, with essentially the same results in the United Kingdom, United States, and Canada. Actually, however, it is difficult to make direct comparisons of the various studies because they differ so much methodologically. Most of the studies used questionnaires or highly structured interviews, and these procedures necessarily limited the kinds of information that could be received. A few generalizations may be made nevertheless. It is apparent that patient behaviors that are associated with the illness are disruptive, but it is not clear that any certain kinds of behaviors are most disruptive. That is, first-rank symptoms (delusions, hallucinations, and thought disorder) and second-rank symptoms (apathy, anhedonia, lack of motivation) appear on the list of burdensome behaviors. What does perhaps stand out is the patient's need for regular and close supervision. This demand on family time and effort was often mentioned, more often than such behaviors as violence and aggressiveness, which are stereotypically viewed as the major problems of living with the mentally ill person. Indeed, these more active behaviors were mentioned, but less often than the patient's passivity, suggesting that the families interviewed were dealing with the chronic condition of mental illness.

Subjective burden. The term *subjective burden* has been used to indicate the impact of living with mental illness on the family member. The experience is presumably stressful, and reactions to this stress have been assessed by several researchers. One of the earliest reports was by Grad and Sainsbury (1968) in their comparison of two psychiatric treatment programs in Great Britain. More than one-half of the family members interviewed believed their own mental health had been affected, with worry about the patient mentioned most often. They also spoke of insomnia, headaches, excessive irritability, and depression.

In the United States, Spaniol et al. (1985) received completed questionnaires from 140 NAMI members. The symptoms of stress that they reported, with the percentage of respondents mentioning a particular item, were anxiety (58%), frustration (58%), worry (56%), sense of burden (55%), depression (48%), grief (47%), fear (44%), and anger (42%). These were symptoms that had increased over the past year; symptoms that had decreased over the past year included shame (21%) and guilt (18%). Hatfield's (1978) sample of NAMI members (*n* = 89) yielded similar results. She found that they reported stress (65%), anxiety (30%), resentment (24%), and grief and depression (22%). These family members went on to say that their experiences with mental illness also had negative consequences for family life and cited increased marital strain (20%), disrupted social life (17%), hardship for siblings (27%), and a disrupted personal life (14%).

Thompson and Doll (1982) questioned family members of patients who had been in three state hospitals in Ohio. They found that 73% of the family members were adversely affected in one or more ways. In particular, these respondents said they felt overloaded (72%), embarrassed (46%), entrapped (42%), and resentful (40%). Fenton et al. (1979) reported that the families of patients in their Montreal psychiatric treatment programs typically were worried about the illness (71%), anxious (68%), fatigued (51%), and depressed (51%).

In a study of relatives of patients with schizophrenia in a first episode, McCreadie et al. (1987) found very high levels of anxiety-based symptoms: 77% were above the caseness level. That the relatives were interviewed when the patient was in crisis undoubtedly contributed to the high levels of distress found; nevertheless, these results strongly suggest that relatives coping with psychiatric crisis should be regarded as a group at risk for stress-related disorders.

Arey and Warheit (1980) did an epidemiological survey of 4,202 adults living in six Florida counties. Randomly selected respondents were asked if they had a family member with serious nervous or emotional problems and what the relationship of the family member was to the respondent. Interviewees were also asked to complete self-report rating scales designed to assess the level of experienced anxiety, depression, and psychosocial dysfunction. The results showed that anxiety, depression, and psychosocial dysfunction were all significantly higher for respondents who had a mentally ill family member than for those who did not; in fact, the level of reported anxiety and depression was twice as high, and the level of psychosocial dysfunction was three times as high. Further analyses of the data indicated that being of low socioeconomic status was associated with higher levels of difficulty: blacks reported more difficulty than whites and women more difficulty than men, and persons living alone with the disturbed person had more problems than those who shared responsibilities with someone else. The highest levels of anxiety, depression, and psychosocial dysfunction were reported by low-income black women. The level of perceived difficulty was also higher in general if more than one mentally ill person was in the home. Anxiety and depression were highest when the mentally ill person was a child, but psychosocial dysfunction was highest when the disturbed person was a parent.

Economic burden.   Several investigators have included measures of economic burden in their studies of the impact of mental illness on the family, but information on this matter has not been gathered in a systematic way. In their random sample of relatives of patients being discharged from three state hospitals, Thompson and Doll (1982) found that 38% of relatives reported experiencing a financial burden and that this burden was higher for families lower on the socioeconomic scale. Holden and Lewine (1982) reported that 32% of NAMI members surveyed said that economic problems were "serious." In all, 74% of their sample reported being affected financially by the mental illness.

Hatfield's (1979) survey of NAMI families showed that 18% wanted help in obtaining relief from financial stress. Lefley (1987b) surveyed mental health professionals who had a mentally ill family member. An attempt was made to estimate costs for hospitalization and treatment exclusive of insurance. Estimates ranged from $300 to $150,000 with a mean of $44,080 during the course of illness. However, many of the respondents, instead of giving a dollar figure, wrote "a great deal." It seems likely that the estimates given greatly underestimate the actual costs of caring for a mentally ill person because only hospitalization and treatment costs were included in estimates. This left out such costs as attorneys' fees for getting the person out of jail, airline tickets used to bring the person back home from far-off places, food, clothing replaced after loss, alternative housing, etc.

Johnson's (1985) survey of NAMI members asked about present housing and willingness to contribute to the cost of alternative housing in the community. Most (77%) said their mentally ill family member was not living at home at the time of the interview, and of this group of respondents, 80% were not satisfied with current arrangements. They were in agreement about what they regarded as adequate residential facilities, and 68% said they would be able to pay part of the cost of such a living arrangement. The amounts suggested ranged from $200 to $600 per month, with a mean of $334.

In a study carried out in the United Kingdom, Hoenig and Hamilton (1969) reported that 30% of families of schizophrenic patients said their financial status had suffered and 7% had lost earnings.

Surveys have been conducted to compare the effects of hospital treatment with community treatment and have included some measure of financial burden on the family. Grad and Sainsbury (1968) compared families of patients in hospital and community programs in a 2-year follow-up. Both groups reported that mental illness had had an impact on the family's financial status owing to reduced work capacity, having to leave work to care for a mentally ill person, and other not-described costs. Furthermore, community care left a greater family burden than hospital care.

It is clear from these survey results that families of the mentally ill are placed under financial stress, but the definitive analysis of the actual financial burden of mental illness on families has not been carried out. Just how much burden there is depends on whether the mentally ill person is the household's principal breadwinner or a dependent child, whether extensive community assistance is available, and the overall financial condition of the family. One of the most illuminating accounts of the economic costs of mental illness is found in the Hinckleys' book (Hinckley et al. 1985) about their son's mental illness and trial after his attack on the president. Even this relatively affluent family was very hard pressed financially by the chain of events.

Parents

As parents were most often the subjects of the surveys reviewed above, their concerns and reactions have already been presented. They do, however, also have some unique concerns. The care of the mentally ill person often falls quite naturally to the parents. Mental illness tends to appear in the late teens and early twenties, a time when most children have just begun to move out of the parental home. Some are away at school, but still financially dependent on parents. With the onset of their illness, this dependency is prolonged. Parents take up the cause of seeking treatment and coping with the mentally ill person's behavior. Among the two commonly heard concerns are questions of guilt ("What did I do to cause this terrible illness?") and of long-term care ("Who will take care of him/her after we're gone?").

Spouses

Spouses of the mentally ill have many problems, many of which center around role performance. Traditionally, the husband's role has been to work and provide financial support for the family and the wife's role has been to manage the household and care for the children. Although the traditional role relationships have undergone major changes in the past two decades, vestiges of them remain. The research of Clausen (1975), Clausen and Huffine (1979), Noh and Turner (1987), Runck (1979), and Rogler and Hollingshead (1965) has been especially helpful in showing how the course of mental illness disrupts family life. With mental illness in a spouse, financial and sexual problems increase and there is a great need to protect children from harm, emotionally as well as physically.

Siblings

Without doubt, this is the neglected group of relatives of the mentally ill. There is little in the literature directly related to the experiences of siblings. Bleuler (1978) has a chapter on siblings in his book on schizophrenia, and siblings were included in his longitudinal research, but studied only as they might contribute to an understanding of the genetics of schizophrenia. Schulz et al. (1982) included siblings in their study of patient and family attitudes about schizophrenia, but their sample was small. They point out that the inheritance of schizophrenia is a troublesome issue for this group. Siblings also worry about their own sanity, dread the day when they may have full responsibility for their mentally ill sibling's care, and often have mixed feelings about the care provided by their parents for the mentally ill family member. They feel left out of what is going on in the family because no one tells them how to understand the disturbed person's behavior. Carlisle (1984) interviewed 20 siblings of schizophrenic or manic-depressive patients and found the same concerns as those mentioned above. Her report is a powerful presentation of the severe impact mental illness has on siblings.

The lack of information about the effect of mental illness on siblings will perhaps be repaired now that a subsection of NAMI made up of siblings has been formed.

Children

There is a substantial literature on the children of the mentally ill, but, with only a few exceptions, it is concerned entirely with the effects on child development of being reared by a mentally ill parent (Mednick et al. 1975; Rice et al. 1971; Sameroff and Zax 1978). These include such child behaviors as performance in school, peer relations, and psychological organization, but it is beyond the scope of this chapter to review this literature.

One of the few studies of adult children of the mentally ill was done by Bleuler (1974, 1978). In his longitudinal study of schizophrenia, he followed the 184 children of 208 schizophrenic parents. At the time of the last follow-up, almost all of these children were adults. Although the principal purpose of the research on these children was to explore genetic relationships, Bleuler came to know the families very well, and he made a number of pertinent observations about the burden of mental illness as experienced by these adult children. He wondered about the neglect of these individuals by mental health professionals, from both clinical and research perspectives. He wrote:

> . . . the principal reason seems to lie in the children themselves. All too often they remain silent about their sufferings and can seldom be moved to discuss them. Even after they have grown up, they much prefer to keep to themselves everything terrible and disagreeable that happened to them. Somehow they consider it a disgrace to have suffered so much misery at the hands of their own parents. It actually happens that the misery of a neglected child, caused by the psychosis of a father or mother, is the cause of ridicule and disgrace, not only at the hands of his schoolmates, but also of people who ought to know better, for instance, his teachers. (Bleuler 1978, p. 405)

Bleuler went on to describe the experiences of some of these children and summarized:

> Many children of schizophrenics have to endure appalling childhoods. Not only do they suffer often, and quite directly, under their sick parents, but often they are entrusted to foster parents who are not by any standards suited to that role. Sometimes a healthy father or mother has little understanding of how to bring up a child unassisted. The children of schizophrenics quite ordinarily exhibit pathological behavior or development during their childhoods that only seldom attain the magnitude of psychoses. In small children especially, fear is at the very forefront of their existence. At times bodily

manifestations of fear dominate the picture. As the child grows older, increasing communication disorders are added to the fear. The children grow shy, inept at human contacts, retiring, sensitive, and either provocative and aggressive or apathetic. Their mood is depressed and unhappy. Often the children withdraw into fantasies and daydreaming. A number of authors combine such personality changes into a general category they call "schizoid." Children may also take on the hallucinatory ideas of their parents, establishing a specific type of folie-a-deux. Of course, not nearly all offspring of schizophrenics experience an adverse childhood development. There are vast numbers of examples that show how even schizophrenic parents can be good parents. Some children learn to distinguish what it is about their father or mother that is peculiar or sick, and what is good and lovable about him or her. Sometimes gifted, warm-hearted spouses are able to nullify all the evil influences of the other partner who is schizophrenic. (Bleuler 1978, pp. 405–406)

One of his subjects seemed to be speaking for many adult children of schizophrenic parents as well as for himself when he said, "When you've been through that . . . you can never really be happy; you can never laugh as others do, you always have to be ashamed of yourself and take care not to break down yourself" (Bleuler 1978, p. 410).

Bleuler's observations poignantly describe the experience of one group of family members who have lived intimately with schizophrenia. He has also noted that for many of these individuals, growing up did not mean leaving this experience behind—as adults they continued to live with their parents, but now as caretakers of their mentally ill parent.

Clausen and Huffine (1979) have called for more research with this group. In their own work, they found the children of the mentally ill were bothered by parental dishonesty ("Like my father hides his liquor, she hides her hallucinations") and by the hallucinatory behavior itself, feeling that they were being shut out of communication with their parent. The children also felt that they were not told about mental illness, especially if the mother was the ill parent; mothers were more apt to provide information if the father was ill. The children also reported that they found it difficult to negotiate with their parents about delusional ideas. Behaviors based on delusions created great uncertainty for the children. Finally, children felt guilty, that they were somehow responsible for the emotional disturbance of their parent.

Other Relatives

The other relatives of the mentally ill, the grandparents, cousins, stepparents, and others, seem not to have been the objects of much specific research. In one study, Wender et al. (1971) found that adoptive parents of children who became schizophrenic showed emotional problems that appeared to be reactive to the adopted child's disturbance. The adoptive parents showed depression, anxiety, and withdrawal, and they felt guilty.

It is apparent from the various NAMI-type surveys that other relatives are frequently involved closely in the care of a mentally ill family member and share in the caretaking burden. Accounts such as that by Vine (1982) make it clear that this involvement is at least as intense and burdensome as that experienced by first-degree relatives.

CONDITIONS AFFECTING LEVEL OF BURDEN

Families of the mentally ill do not have a uniform experience of burden when caring for the ill person. All of the surveys show a considerable range of experience on virtually all questions asked. It is, therefore, more important to ask under what circumstances the burden is great than to ask the general question of whether there is a burden.

Characteristics of the Mentally Ill Person

The strikingly consistent pattern of female respondents about male mentally ill offspring raises a question as to whether there are differences in the burden experienced by the family as a function of sex of the mentally ill person. Perhaps relatives of male patients have joined NAMI and similar organizations because male patients are more difficult. For a partial answer to this question, it is necessary to turn to the few studies that have reported sex differences in burden. Unfortunately, most of the researchers who could have provided answers to this question have been silent on the issue. Only three studies have reported on the relationship between burden and sex of the mentally ill family member. Grad and Sainsbury (1968) and Thompson and Doll (1982) found no sex differences, and Hoenig and Hamilton (1969) found that male patients presented a greater burden. On the basis of this very limited information, little can be said. If it is assumed that the other researchers have not commented on the issue because they have not found sex differences, then it might be concluded tentatively that the sex of the mentally ill person is not an important contributor to family burden.

Several studies have shown that the level of symptoms is highly related to the amount of burden felt; that is, if the patient is highly disturbed, caretaking is more difficult for the family members. Thompson and Doll (1982) surveyed relatives of patients recently discharged from three Ohio state hospitals. They found that patient sex, age, and social class were not related to the amount of burden experienced by the family members. The psychiatric condition of the patient was significantly related to burden. With higher levels of disturbance, family members were more likely to report feeling embarrassed, overloaded, trapped, and resentful. Herz et al. (1976) found measures of burden to be related to such patient behaviors as belligerence, unpleasantness, disorganization, and impaired reality testing. These results were essentially confirmed by a similar study carried out by Potasznik and Nelson (1984). They found that both objective and subjective burden were related to level of patient symptomatology. McCreadie et al. (1987) also found a high correlation between patients' disturbance and relatives' anxiety in a study of first-episode patients.

Hospital or Community Care

Deinstitutionalization has created many problems, not the least of which is the increased burden placed on families. In a sense, much of the burden described earlier is a product of deinstitutionalization. However, there has been little research on differences in burden found for patients maintained in the community versus those kept in hospitals. Of the studies that have made this comparison, Grad and Sainsbury (1968) in England found greater burden for families of community-treated patients, but more recent research has found either no differences between groups or less burden for families of the community-treated group. Grad and Sainsbury (1968) did a 24-month follow-up comparison of families of patients treated largely in the community with families of patients who were treated in hospitals. They concluded that community care created a greater burden; families had more problems to contend with. A similar study was conducted in New York by Herz et al. (1976), who compared standard inpatient treatment followed by discharge when the therapists believed the patient was ready, brief hospitalization followed by transitional day care, and brief hospitalization with discharge to the community. Family members reported high levels of burden in general, but these were higher for the brief hospitalization groups when interviewed 3 weeks after release from the hospital. At this time, most of the standard inpatient group was still in the hospital. At 24 weeks, there were no differences between groups on measures of burden, but about one-fourth of all families believed the patient had come home too soon.

Fenton et al. (1979) compared home- and hospital-treated patients in Quebec. When family burden was assessed as long as a year after hospital discharge, they found no differences between groups. The lack of difference was due, according to the authors, to the availability of adequate support services to both groups.

In a Wisconsin study by Test and Stein (1980), patients were treated in the community or in the hospital, and family burden was assessed 1 month and 4 months after the patient entered the project. The groups did not differ at 1 month, and at 4 months, the community-group families reported a significant decrease in burden. This approach was replicated in Australia by Reynolds and Hoult (1984). At the 12-month interview, family burden did not differ significantly between groups. Although levels of burden remained fairly high for both groups, the community-group families reported very high levels of satisfaction with the services received.

These studies suggest that it is not whether a patient is treated in a hospital or in the community per se that is important for family burden, but it is the presence of supportive services that makes a difference. There is one warning note, however: the one study that reported higher levels of burden for family members when community treatment was emphasized was the only one that followed families as long as 2 years. As Fenton et al. (1979) have noted, the beneficial effects of community care tend to diminish over time. If care is not continued, treatment gains disappear, and, one would expect, family burden would again increase.

Time

Several studies of experienced burden have found that the number of relatives who report high levels of burden declines with time (Fenton et al. 1979; Gibbons et al. 1984; Grad and Sainsbury 1968; Smith 1969; Test and Stein 1980). Other studies, however, have shown continuing burden and increasing stress over time (Herz et al. 1976; Hoenig and Hamilton 1969; Noh and Turner 1987; Spaniol et al. 1984). Again, the warning that burden may increase when professional care is discontinued should be heeded.

Presence of Support Networks

Potasznik and Nelson (1984) looked at the burden experienced by families as a function of kinds and extensiveness of social networks utilized. They found that the sense of burden was lower if the family members were involved with small, dense social networks, if these network experiences were seen as satisfying, and if their spouse was helpful in caring for the patient. Involvement in a self-help group was especially important in reducing burden.

Table 1.   Family members' (n = 43) mean level of satisfaction with information received from mental health professionals

How to obtain a commitment	2.74 (4)
Diagnosis	2.60 (12)
Management of medications	2.45 (5)
How to obtain help in a crisis	2.43 (6)
How to locate residential care	2.37 (11)
How to obtain respite care	2.32 (24)
How to respond to delusions, etc.	2.24 (14)
Cause of mental illness	2.24 (5)
Obtaining SSI or SSDI	2.17 (8)
How to cope with bizarre behavior	1.94 (10)
How to manage withdrawn behavior	1.77 (13)
How to cope with violence	1.69 (14)

Note.   Values are based on a 5-point scale, with 5 indicating very satisfied. Issues are ranked from most to least satisfied. Number of respondents with no experience in that particular matter is shown in parentheses.
SSI = supplemental security income. SSDI = social security disability income.
Source.   Data are from Johnson 1985.

Experiences With Mental Health Providers

The severe problems caused by mental illness make it virtually inevitable that those closely associated with the mentally ill will have to seek the help of professionals. A large and diverse group of professionals are available to provide services, in both private and public sectors. They represent many different occupational groups, and they hold such widely differing ideologies that it is not clear what they have in common. With this diversity, it is difficult to be precise about the experiences family members have with professionals. There have been, however, several surveys of family members' reactions to professionals.

Johnson (1985) did a telephone survey of members of a mental health advocacy group and had 43 completed interviews. One part of this survey dealt with satisfaction with mental health services. One set of questions were about satisfaction with information received. Respondents were to rate their satisfaction on a 5-point scale with 5 indicating "very satisfied." They were also asked to indicate whether they had experience with the issue. The most remarkable result of the survey was that families were not very satisfied with information received from professionals (Table 1). The average ratings shown in Table 1 indicate that the level of satisfaction is, at best, between "fairly satisfied" and "not at all satisfied," and for kinds of information, satisfaction is very low. Quite clearly, family members have been given

Table 2. Family members' (n = 43) mean level of satisfaction with mental health services

Medical examination	3.00 (6)
Psychological evaluation	2.97 (4)
Social skills training	2.95 (17)
Day hospital program	2.90 (33)
Individual psychotherapy	2.80 (8)
Group therapy	2.70 (16)
Neurological evaluation	2.44 (16)
Vocational rehabilitation	2.38 (18)
Medication	2.36 (3)
Community mental health center referral	2.22 (16)
Family therapy	2.21 (9)
Case management	1.96 (19)
Hospital discharge planning	1.78 (11)

Note. Values are based on a 5-point scale, with 5 indicating very satisfied. Services are listed from most to least satisfactory. Number of respondents with no experience in that particular matter is shown in parentheses.
Source. Data are from Johnson 1985.

little or no help in dealing with psychotic behaviors, but even for such basic questions as the diagnosis of the family member, clear and meaningful information has not been provided.

A similar question was asked about satisfaction with services received, and again, respondents were asked to rate their satisfaction on a 5-point scale (Table 2). The ratings show a wider range of satisfaction than for ratings for information received, but again the most noteworthy feature is the low level of satisfaction with mental health services. It is also important to consider how often family members report having had no experience with a particular service. In some instances, this is not surprising because the service may not be necessary in all cases, but when 19 of 43 families had no experience with case management, something is seriously wrong with the system. It is also worth noting that "hospital discharge planning" appears at the bottom of the ranking of satisfaction: most family members were very dissatisfied with how this was handled. At the other end of the scale, we see that professionals are able to provide some services in a satisfactory way; they seem to do best on examinations.

Family members were also asked to rate their overall satisfaction with the rehabilitative care their family member is receiving at the present time. Once again, the level of satisfaction is low. Fifty-eight percent said they were not satisfied, 17% thought the treatment was fairly good, and only 26% were completely satisfied. With such a low level of satisfaction, it might be wondered whether respondents had

Table 3. Number of mentions of good or bad experience with type of mental health professional or service by family members of mentally ill patients (n = 43)

Good experience		Bad experience	
Psychiatrists	25	Psychiatrists	27
Public facilities	13	Public facilities	21
Professionals, general	13	Professionals, general	8
Psychologists	7	Private facilities	3
Social workers	6	Social workers	2
Private facilities	1	Administrators, general	2
Administrators, general	1	Psychologists	1
		Police	1

Note. Results are shown in rank order of number of mentions.
Source. Data are from Johnson 1985.

ever taken action to remove their family member from an unsatisfactory situation. Sixteen percent had removed him or her from an unsatisfactory situation, 16% had removed him or her from an alternative care home, 21% had taken him or her out of a hospital, and 23% had "fired" their doctor.

Finally, respondents were asked to tell about two especially good experiences they had had with professional mental health workers and then to tell about two especially bad experiences (Table 3). The results show how important the medical doctor is to family members in the treatment of serious mental disorders. Psychiatrists were praised and criticized at a very high rate, and unfortunately, the numbers do not convey the strength of feeling that family members have about mental health professionals, feelings that may be positive or negative.

The Spaniol et al. (1984) survey of NAMI members found that family members were divided in their satisfaction with mental health services: 45% were satisfied and another 45% were dissatisfied. Dissatisfaction was greatest with social rehabilitation, vocational rehabilitation, individual therapy, and drug medication. Drug medication and individual psychotherapy also received relatively high satisfaction ratings, along with hospitalization. Family members were also dissatisfied with treatment coordination, practical advice, information about the illness, emotional support, and referral. They were relatively satisfied with the professionals' attitudes toward the mentally ill person and family member.

Hatfield (1979) also surveyed NAMI members about the value of help received from mental health professionals and other persons in coping with mental illness in the family. Services provided by professionals such as individual, group, or family therapy, although reported as helpful by about one-half of the respondents, received much lower ratings than did such resources as parents of other schizophrenic patients, friends, and relatives.

It may be of particular interest to know what mental health professionals with mentally ill family members think about the services provided by mental health professionals. All mental health professions were represented in a survey carried out by Lefley (1987b), and the respondents were siblings (38%), parents (30%), or children (21%) of a mentally ill person. Asked to rate their perceptions of the behavior of professionals toward the family of the mentally ill person, respondents gave professionals few high marks. Professionals were rated low especially on "instruct families in how to try to prevent recurrence of psychotic episodes," "provide adequate information on how to manage bizarre or disruptive behavior," and "provide adequate information about nature of illness or disorder." Relatively positive ratings were given for "instruct families in medication side effects," "treat families with warmth and compassion," and "recognize families in pain over illness of loved ones." On activities carried out by professionals, medical services such as chemotherapy and other somatic therapies received highest ratings. The psychotherapies, including family therapy, pastoral counseling, and marital therapy, were given much lower ratings on "helpfulness." In general, it appears that mental health professionals who have mentally ill family members have reacted in about the same way to the mental health professionals they have encountered as have nonprofessional family members.

Respondents to the survey of NAMI members conducted by Holden and Lewine (1982) also reported a high level of dissatisfaction with the services provided by mental health professionals. Of the 203 respondents, 78% said they were "generally dissatisfied" or "very dissatisfied." Mental health professionals were the persons most often consulted to help in a crisis, but after working with the professionals, families often said they felt "frustrated." Another often-reported feeling was a sense of powerlessness. As already noted, families experience a sense of helplessness in attempting to cope with mental illness, and, when dealing with professionals, they find this feeling of powerlessness is again present. Families reported that professionals were least helpful in directing them to community resources such as housing and vocational help. They also said that there was little follow-up on medication prescriptions. Little guidance was offered about how to handle bizarre or delusional behaviors. Most (68%) were told the mentally ill person's diagnosis within 2 years of first hospitalization, but little explanation of the meaning of the diagnosis was given.

Howe (1985) has directed attention to the special problems created for families by family therapists. She reported that families say they have been pressured to attend family therapy sessions, and that no excuses were allowed for not having the entire family present for the sessions. This coercion has included telling family members that no further services will be available for the mentally ill family member unless the family participates in family therapy. Furthermore, it is the common experience of families that they have been severely abused by family therapists—blamed for causing the mentally ill person's illness and told that the mentally ill person is disturbed primarily because the family will not face up to internal family problems. Considering the conclusions of Terkelsen's (1983) review of the effectiveness of family therapy with schizophrenic patients—there is no evidence that it is effective—one wonders why family therapy is even part of the treatment plan.

The dissatisfaction with mental health professionals has been found in all of the studies of families associated with advocacy groups. It is so uniform and intense that professionals must become aware of these feelings and modify their behavior if they are to carry out their own work effectively. It must be pointed out, however, that not all surveys of families have yielded high levels of dissatisfaction. In fact, a rather different picture is seen if studies of satisfaction with particular treatment programs are reviewed. Hoenig and Hamilton (1969) pointed out that despite high levels of burden experienced, family members in their study of two treatment programs in the United Kingdom reported general satisfaction (69%) with the services received. Only 9% had "serious complaints." The authors noted that the dissatisfactions that were mentioned by family members had to do with feeling that when the patient was released to them from the hospital they were left to fend on their own. The authors also suggested that the relatively high level of satisfaction stemmed from the ready availability of services to patients and families.

Grella and Grusky (1989) investigated relatives' satisfaction with services in a small sample of families in the American Northwest. They found that two-thirds were "less than satisfied," but that satisfaction increased when they had much contact with case managers.

Herz et al. (1976) also reported that family members were "generally positive" toward their programs. These programs, both inpatient and outpatient, included active support of families by the staff. The major complaint was that patients were sent home from the hospital too soon.

Reynolds and Hoult (1984) compared an in-community treatment program that was based on that developed by Stein and Test (1980) with standard hospital care and aftercare. The community program included a great deal of contact with relatives, much more than was received by families of patients in the standard program. One year after intake, families were asked how satisfied they were with various aspects of treatment. The two groups of relatives differed significantly on all items, and most of the community program relatives were satisfied with the amount of treatment or care (90%), amount of supervision (83%), support and help (81%), advice and information (71%), and medication (71%). By contrast, fewer than half of the standard program relatives were satisfied with the services received on these items.

Much the same result was obtained by Falloon et al. (1984) in their survey of satisfaction with a family management training program compared with an individual psychotherapy control group. Both groups of families were recipients of a considerable amount of staff attention, and even though the family management group was the specific target of family-oriented training, both groups of relatives expressed high levels of satisfaction with the services received. In fact, it appears that virtually all participants of both groups were satisfied. There were few expressions of dissatisfaction at any time.

These surveys of satisfaction with specific programs indicate that dissatisfaction is not merely a characteristic of the relatives of the mentally ill. They cannot be viewed as a complaining, dysfunctional group of people. On the contrary, Creer and Wing (1975) remarked on how little complaining they did considering the burden that they had to carry. If family members are granted consideration by professionals and given access to an array of appropriate services, they readily express satisfaction with the services and are grateful to the mental health professionals who provided them.

DIFFERENTIAL ASSESSMENT OF FAMILY NEEDS
BY PROFESSIONALS AND FAMILIES

When professionals were asked if family members were satisfied with their services, they responded that the great majority (82%) were (Spaniol et al. 1984). In this same survey, professionals also believed that families were satisfied with the many specific services provided. These findings are in sharp contrast with the results of surveys of family members themselves. The contrast suggests a serious lack of communication about consumer issues. As Creer and Wing (1975) stated, family members rarely complain. Why they do not does not seem to have been the subject of research, but the reasons are not obscure: they trust professionals, they are often in despair and are inclined to blame themselves for things that go wrong, and they are afraid that if they complain they will lose services on which they are desperately dependent.

Interpretation of Conflict

Conflict between professionals and family members seems to occur quite frequently. In one form, a family member has reason to doubt that treatment is being carried out effectively or that the mentally ill person is not being treated humanely. Complaints are made and action is requested. In some instances, if action is not taken by the professionals directly responsible, the requests are taken to higher authorities. Family members see this kind of action on their part as unfortunately necessary to repair the failures of professionals. Professionals, on the other hand, see this as unwarranted usurpation of their authority. Harbin (1978) has warned that this may be manipulative and that administrators should be aware that such family behaviors may be a form of acting out in order to avoid making necessary changes in the family system.

Another form of conflict arises over the acceptability of specific treatment forms. Howe (1985) pointed out that families often have serious and substantial reasons for not wanting to participate in treatment that to them seems to have little to do with the needed treatment of the mentally ill person. A difference in treatment ideologies may be part of the problem (Jones and Graybill 1984), but different assessments of family resources are also often involved. For example, families are sometimes told that they must participate as an entire family in family therapy sessions for an unspecified period of time. Families reply that they cannot meet at the times set because of work, school, or other demands on their time. This action is interpreted by some professionals, especially those with a family systems orientation, as being "resistance to systemic change" (Stratton and Seman 1982). The concept of resistance has been used often by professionals to justify their own behaviors and to deprecate those of patients and families. It seems possible that the concept could also be used by family members to serve their own purposes, that is, the behaviors of some professionals could be interpreted as resistance. But whether used by professionals or families, the concept seems to be used more in a pejorative than a therapeutic sense, with its main function being to define the limits of power in the therapy relationship.

Issue of Dysfunctional Families

Some mental health professionals either assume or find that virtually all families of the mentally ill are inept and dysfunctional. Munro (1985) referred to the "pathology in the entire system" when referring to the families of the mentally ill. The recent report by Spitzer et al. (1982) exemplifies this view. They studied 79 families of patients admitted for the first time to the University of Iowa medical school hospital. The families were interviewed at length at admission, and patients were followed up 10 years later. Families were typed according to their level of expected performance for the patient and their propensity for action. Families were rated as either high or low on these two dimensions, yielding four types of families. They added subtypes, making use of other information such as interpersonal style and attitudes toward the concepts and practices of mental health professionals. Without reviewing their research, what is of interest here are the terms they used to characterize the various types of families: assertives, altercasters, authoritarians, stoics, poltroons, pacifists, stumblers, and do-nothings. Many of the terms are obviously pejorative, and even the terms that on the surface are not, when defined also are revealed as negative toward family members. Furthermore, in none of the 12 cases cited to illustrate their typology are family members presented in a positive light. The authors were apparently unable to find anything positive to say about the attempts of family members to cope with the difficulties presented by mental illness.

Another use of typologies of families (Krajewski and Harbin 1982) presents the families in an equally negative way. This typology is simple; it is comprised of only three kinds of family reactions to mental illness: overinvolved, underinvolved, and pseudoinvolved. The authors did say, however, that this typology includes only those families who have not made "legitimate" interventions with the hospital staff. There was no further discussion of these legitimate behaviors, and no case studies of these families were presented. For the types of family reactions discussed, all of the cases offered are negative toward family members. Interestingly, one of the chief areas of conflict between families and staff had to do with family participation in family therapy—apparently some families objected to this form of involvement.

The studies discussed above were selected only because they seemed to represent a general point of view about families in the mental health professions. In unpublished form, for example, in clinical case conferences, families are frequently described in less gentle terms.

Spaniol et al. (1984) found that what professionals most often mentioned when asked what families needed was family therapy. The belief that families are dysfunctional is pervasive.

Role of Mental Health Ideologies

In no other area of treatment for illness have families of the ill been such objects of contempt and scathing criticism by professionals as have the families of the mentally ill. Parents of autistic children and parents of schizophrenic persons have been especially harshly treated. The bases of this treatment in psychoanalytic theory and more recently in family therapy theory have been reviewed many times and need not be repeated here (Johnson 1984; Terkelsen 1983). It is important to note that the actions of professionals who have been guided by these theories have tended to divide families and to keep families ignorant and powerless. Blame has been used to maintain the professional in power. Family members have been made to feel guilty for causing the illness, whether intentionally or not. One consequence is that by viewing families as malevolent, or incompetent, professionals have distanced themselves from the families.

To paraphrase Bleuler (1978) when he wrote of the children of the mentally ill, their "misery . . . is the cause of ridicule and disgrace . . . by the people who ought to know better, for instance, the professionals." Indeed, mental health professionals "ought to know better," but they are guided by theory, and the theories have had a negative view of family members. There may be some change in this; certainly there is if one uses current scientific journals as an indicator, in which one can detect within psychiatry a change toward a greater biological emphasis and within clinical psychology a greater emphasis on cognitive behavioral theories of mental disorder, neither of which includes blame of family members as an important part of its etiological system. Nevertheless, a vast number of mental health professionals are still influenced by family-blaming psychodynamic and family therapy ideologies.

WHAT FAMILIES WANT FROM PROFESSIONALS

The overriding concern of family members—their highest priority wish—is that professionals provide effective treatment for the mentally ill person. Early in the treatment process, the wish is for a cure, a return to normality, but as the mental illness continues, family members accept the mental illness and wish for improvement if not cure. At the second level of priority, what they want may be inferred from the kinds of dissatisfaction that they have expressed toward the services of professionals. In short, because they know that a major part of the burden of caring for the mentally ill person will fall on them, they want to be able to cope better. The surveys of family members have been consistent in finding the following wants for family members (Johnson 1985; Leavitt 1975; Lefley 1987a, 1987b; Smets 1982; Spaniol et al. 1984).

1. *Information.* Family members want to know more about the cause
    of the disorder, the nature of the illness, and how to prevent
    relapse. They want specific information on the role of medication
    in treatment, what are the common side effects, and how to help
    the patient to take medication as prescribed. They also want to
    know how to deal with strange, delusional behaviors and how to
    prevent attacks against family members. They also need infor-
    mation about supplemental security income and vocational and
    other community rehabilitation services.
2. *Access to resources.* Families want to be able to obtain services when
    they are needed. This includes having effective information and
    referral services available.
3. *Continuity of care.* A major fear of families is that professionals
    will simply "dump" the family member on them or onto the com-
    munity at large. They want professionals to provide continuity
    for what they know is a very long-term rehabilitation process.
4. *Respect and understanding.* Family members want professionals to
    recognize that they are intelligent, able individuals who can ben-
    efit from information. They want to be treated with compassion
    and understanding. They want to be able to talk with the profes-
    sional and know that their concerns, ideas, and feelings have been
    heard.

COPING AND ADAPTATION SKILLS

Whether the family members of the mentally ill are viewed as
relatives of the mentally ill person and as part of a family system that
may serve as a resource for the mentally ill member or as persons in
their own right, efforts should be made to see that they retain their
mental health, competence, and economic viability. If this point of
view is adopted, then the issue of prevention is raised. Much has been
made of the need to offer a wide range of preventive services, and
there has been some misunderstanding about what targets this might
include. Attention has often been directed at preventing the onset of
such disorders as schizophrenia, and critics have said that this is only
a dream until the cause of schizophrenia is known. Prevention, however, may be directed at other problems, including those reported by
the families of patients with mental illnesses for which the cause is
now at least partially known. By reducing the burden of living with
mental illness, such stress disorders as depression and anxiety could
be alleviated.

CONDITIONS FOR MINIMIZING IMPACT

The burden of coping with mental illness can be eased by means that are now available. There are three general ways that have been demonstrated through research to be effective in reducing the burden on families of mental illness—support networks, psychiatric services, and family management training.

Networks

For many people, the most significant advance in psychiatry in recent decades has been the growth of self-help and advocacy groups. The self-help revolution began in the 1930s when Alcoholics Anonymous was formed. Other groups of distressed people were slow in adopting the self-help model, but today there are such groups for nearly every medical and psychological condition. Similar self-help and advocacy groups for families of the mentally ill were formed about a dozen years ago in California, but the national organization was formed only 6 years ago. Its growth in such a short period has been phenomenal.

Many accounts of the usefulness of these groups exist, but they are largely anecdotal; systematic research on the effectiveness is lacking for all self-help groups, including Alcoholics Anonymous. There is, however, evidence that social support is helpful in alleviating stress. Potasznik and Nelson (1984) found that experienced burden was less when parents of the mentally ill reported that "their networks are small and dense, when they are satisfied with the support of their total network and the self-help group, and when their spouses spend considerable time with the patient" (p. 599).

Psychiatric Services

Inasmuch as experienced burden is related to the severity of the patient's symptomatology, it might be expected that psychiatric services that are effective in relieving symptoms would be effective in relieving family burden. This is undoubtedly true, judging from the evidence reviewed above that some programs have improved patient status and reduced burden. What may be very important in this, however, is that effective treatment does more than reduce first-rank symptoms—those of delusions, hallucinations, and thought disorder—the symptoms that seem most susceptible to treatment by the antipsychotic medications. Families have reported as much burden from patient apathy, listlessness, and lack of feeling—the second-rank symptoms—and treatment for these symptoms calls for extensive psychosocial programming.

Services that have been provided especially to families who have caretaking responsibilities have been successful in reducing burden and/or reducing relapse rates. Examples are those by Grad and Sainsbury (1968), Smith (1969), and Pasamanick et al. (1967). Comprehensive community programs that have made special efforts to provide information and other resources to families (Reynolds and Hoult 1984; Test and Stein 1980) have also demonstrated that family burden can be reduced.

Family Management Training

The idea that if families are to be caretakers of their mentally ill members they should receive specific, detailed training for the task is quite new and still not widely applied. The work of Vaughn and Leff (1976) in London, Anderson et al. (1986) in Pittsburgh, Falloon et al. (1984) in southern California, and Tarrier et al. (1988) in Manchester has shown that relapse rates can be reduced substantially with this kind of training. Furthermore, other aspects of patient behavior, such as time in work, training, or school, are improved and symptoms are reduced. Of importance for this review is that family burden is also reduced and satisfaction with the program is high (Falloon et al. 1984). These family training programs are too complex and extensive to be described here, but they include all of the elements mentioned above in the section on what family members want from professionals. There has been some controversy about the utility of family management training for families of the mentally ill in general; one position is that families should not have major caretaking responsibilities for mentally ill family members on a continuing or permanent basis. Family management training includes, however, elements that are so useful to family members as they try to understand and cope with mental illness that it may be of benefit to families, and patients, whether or not the patient lives with the family.

SUMMARY AND CONCLUSIONS

Surveys of families of the adult mentally ill were reviewed to assess the extent to which families were burdened by having a mentally ill person in the family. The results were quite consistent: families feel they are heavily burdened by a wide range of behaviors of the mentally ill person. Family life is disrupted, great demands are made for supervision of the mentally ill person, and the economic costs are great. Furthermore, it is clear that living with mental illness places stresses on family members that lead to feelings of depression, anxiety, fear, and helplessness. Burden does not seem to be affected by the sex of the mentally ill person, but is related to how disturbed the person is. Furthermore, burden is higher when psychiatric services are inadequate.

Family members have expressed great dissatisfaction with the services provided by mental health professionals. However, when families are provided with resources they need to cope with mental illness and when the mentally ill person is receiving effective care, high levels of satisfaction are reported. Professionals surveyed believed that families were typically satisfied with services and that what they needed most was family therapy. Evidence was presented that professionals still view families of the mentally ill as dysfunctional and as a hindrance to therapeutic progress.

Families want an array of resources, assurance of continuity of care, and respect and consideration from professionals. There is evidence that some treatment programs do provide these wants and that they have been successful in improving the condition of patients and, concomitantly, reducing family burden and increasing family satisfaction.

In reading the survey results presented and comparing them with the content of conversations with many parents, siblings, children, and other relatives of the mentally ill, one has the impression that the surveys underestimate the burden of mental illness. Families seem incredibly tolerant of wildly deviant and demanding behaviors and rarely complain. They recognize that the person who is so devastated by mental illness is still the person they have long known and loved. They know this person needs help and want to provide it, but nothing in their life, or in the life of the family, has prepared them for this ongoing emergency. Family members, nevertheless, continue to cope as well as they can, often becoming victims of the accumulating stresses. They are puzzled and angered by the behavior of mental health professionals toward them, but until recently, with the advent of NAMI, have not had a means to present their concerns to professionals in a way that would be heard. The review has suggested a number of recommendations for further research and action.

The surveys were all, with the exception of that by Arey and Warheit (1980), based on nonrepresentative samples, and as a consequence, it is not known what the burden of mental illness is for segments of the population who have not been surveyed. Representative research is necessary.

The work on subjective burden is revealing, but rather superficial. In none of the studies was there a searching examination of the psychological or physical condition of the people who have lived with mental illness for various lengths of time. The criticism of superficiality also applies to the surveys of economic costs to families and to the kinds of behaviors that are most burdensome. A functional analysis of the behaviors of the mentally ill and the impact on family members is needed.

Some family members, notably siblings and adult children of the mentally ill, have been virtually ignored by the survey researchers. More should be known about the impact of mental illness on these people. The provision of help to family members as a primary preventive effort seems well worthwhile. The social costs of the burden of mental illness must be great, and it now appears that preventive means are available and waiting for application.

There have been numerous pleas to view the family as an ally, not an adversary (Hatfield 1979; Johnson 1984; Weinstein 1982), but it is apparent that this goal has not yet been achieved. The frustration that family members and professionals seem to have with each other is undoubtedly a function of the great frustration presented by mental illness in itself given our present state of knowledge, but ideological differences also contribute. Ideologies that place blame on families can only foster the adversary relationship, and family members would prefer that these ideologies be relegated to obsolescence. But can ideologies that have been acquired through long years of training and practice be dropped so easily? Apparently not. They can, perhaps, be modified in such ways that they are made more appropriate for the problem of mental illness. Beels and McFarlane (1982) have reviewed the usefulness of family therapies in the treatment of schizophrenia and have suggested that this issue of appropriateness be considered seriously; that is, a certain form of family therapy may not be appropriate for chronic conditions, but may be helpful during acute phases of a disorder. Much research needs to be done on this broad topic.

Finally, the central point of this review is that the families of the mentally ill need to be viewed in a new way. Instead of viewing them as passive or dysfunctional or oppositional, the evidence indicates that they should be seen as active copers who may have limited resources for dealing with highly unusual circumstances (Hatfield and Lefley 1987). Emphasis should be placed on the constructive aspects of their efforts. Their strengths should be assessed and utilized. They should be given resources to change their own condition from one of helplessness to one of competence.

REFERENCES

Anderson CM, Reiss DJ, Hogarty GE: Schizophrenia and the Family. New York, Guilford, 1986

Arey S, Warheit GJ: Psychosocial costs of living with psychologically disturbed family members, in The Social Consequences of Psychiatric Illness. Edited by Robins L, Clayton P, Wing JK. New York, Brunner/Mazel, 1980, pp 158–175

Bateson G, Jackson DD, Haley J, et al: Toward a theory of schizophrenia. Behav Sci 1:251–264, 1956

Beels CC, McFarlane WR: Family treatments of schizophrenia: background and state of the art. Hosp Community Psychiatry 33:541–550, 1982

Bleuler M: The offspring of schizophrenics. Schizophr Bull 8:93–107, 1974

Bleuler M: The Schizophrenic Disorders. New Haven, CT, Yale University Press, 1978

Brown GW, Bone M, Dalison M, et al: Schizophrenia and Social Care. London, Oxford University Press, 1966

Carlisle W: Siblings of the Mentally Ill. Saratoga, CA, R & E Publishers, 1984

Clausen JA: The impact of mental illness: a twenty-year follow-up, in Life History Research in Psychopathology, Vol 4, 2nd Edition. Edited by Wirt RD, Winokur G, Roff M. Baltimore, MD, Williams & Wilkins, 1975

Clausen JA, Huffine CL: The impact of parental mental illness on children, in Research in Community Mental Health. Edited by Simmons R. Greenwich, CT, JAI Press, 1979

Creer C, Wing JK: Living with a schizophrenic patient. Br J Hosp Med 14:73–82, 1975

Falloon IRH, Boyd JL, McGill CW: Family Care of Schizophrenia. New York, Guilford, 1984

Fenton FR, Tessier L, Struening EL: A comparative trial of home and hospital psychiatric care: one year follow-up. Arch Gen Psychiatry 36:1073–1079, 1979

Fromm-Reichman F: Notes on the development of treatment of schizophrenics by psychoanalytic psychotherapy. Psychiatry 11:263–273, 1948

Gibbons JS, Horn SH, Powell JM, et al: Schizophrenic patients and their families: a survey in a psychiatric service based on a DGH unit. Br J Psychiatry 144:70–77, 1984

Goldman HH: Mental illness and family burden: a public health perspective. Hosp Community Psychiatry 33:557–559, 1982

Grad J, Sainsbury P: The effects that patients have on their families in a community care and a control psychiatric service: a two-year follow-up. Br J Psychiatry 114:265–278, 1968

Grella CE, Grusky O: Families of the seriously mentally ill and their satisfaction with services. Hosp Community Psychiatry 40:831–835, 1989

Harbin HT: Families and hospitals: collusion or cooperation? Am J Psychiatry 135:1496–1499, 1978

Hatfield AB: Psychological costs of schizophrenia to the family. Social Work 23:355–359, 1978

Hatfield AB: Help-seeking behavior in families of schizophrenics. Am J Community Psychol 7:563–569, 1979

Hatfield AB, Lefley HP: Families of the Mentally Ill: Coping and Adaptation. New York, Guilford, 1987

Hatfield AB, Farrell E, Starr S: The family's perspective on the homeless, in The Homeless Mentally Ill. Edited by Lamb HR. Washington, DC, American Psychiatric Press, 1984, pp 279–300

Herz MI, Endicott J, Spitzer RL: Brief versus standard hospitalization: the families. Am J Psychiatry 133:795–801, 1976

Hinckley J, Hinckley J, Sherrill E: Breaking Points. Grand Rapids, MI, Chosen Books, 1985

Hoenig J: The schizophrenic patient at home. Acta Psychiatr Scand 50:297–308, 1974

Hoenig J, Hamilton M: The desegregation of the mentally ill. London, Routledge & Kegan Paul, 1969

Holden DF, Lewine RRJ: How families evaluate mental health professionals, resources and effects of illness. Schizophr Bull 8:626–633, 1982

Howe C: Responding to families of mentally ill children and youth. Paper presented at the 23rd Annual Child Psychiatry Forum, Richmond, VA, 1985

Johnson DL: The needs of the chronically mentally ill: as seen by the consumer, in The Chronically Mentally Ill: Research and Services. Edited by Mirabi M. New York, SP Medical & Scientific Books, 1984

Johnson DL: Citizens' experiences with the mental health system. Citizens Alliance for the Mentally Ill Newsletter, February 1985, pp 2, 3

Jones ME, Graybill D: Attitude similarity and satisfaction of family members of schizophrenics with services of professionals. J Clin Psychol 40:391–393, 1984

Krajewski T, Harbin HT: The family changes the hospital? in The Psychiatric Hospital and the Family. Edited by Harbin HT. New York, SP Medical & Scientific Books, 1982, pp 143–154

Kreisman DE, Joy VD: Family response to the mental illness of a relative: a review of the literature. Schizophr Bull 10:34–57, 1974

Lamb HR, Oliphant E: Schizophrenia through the eyes of families. Hosp Community Psychiatry 29:803–806, 1978

Leavitt M: The discharge crisis: the experience of families of psychiatric patients. Nurs Res 24:33–40, 1975

Lefley HP: The family's response to mental illness in a relative, in Families of the Mentally Ill: Meeting the Challenges (New Directions for Mental Health Services, No 34). Edited by Hatfield AB. San Francisco, CA, Jossey-Bass, 1987a, pp 3–21

Lefley HP: Impact of mental illness in families of mental health professionals. J Nerv Ment Dis 175:613–619, 1987b

Lidz RW, Lidz T: The family environment of schizophrenic patients. Am J Psychiatry 106:332–345, 1949

Mandelbrote B, Folkard S: Some factors related to outcome and social adjustment in schizophrenia. Acta Psychiatr Scand 37:223–235, 1961

McCreadie RG, Wiles DH, Moore JW, et al: The Scottish first episode schizophrenia study, IV: psychiatric and social impact on relatives. Br J Psychiatry 150:340–344, 1987

Mednick S, Schulsinger H, Schulsinger F: Schizophrenia in children of schizophrenic mothers, in Child Personality and Psychopathology, Vol 2. Edited
by Davids A. New York, John Wiley, 1975

Minkoff K: A map of chronic mental patients, in The Chronic Mental Patient.
Edited by Talbott JA. Washington, DC, American Psychiatric Press, 1978

Munro JD: Counseling severely dysfunctional families of mentally and physically disabled persons. Clinical Social Work Journal 13:18–31, 1985

Myers JK, Weissman MM, Tischler GL, et al: Six-month prevalence of psychiatric disorder in three communities. Arch Gen Psychiatry 41:959–
967, 1984

Noh S, Turner RJ: Living with psychiatric patients: implications for the mental health of family members. Soc Sci Med 25:263–271, 1987

Pasamanick B, Scarpitti FR, Dinitz S: Schizophrenics in the Community: An
Experimental Study of the Prevention of Hospitalization. New York,
Appleton-Century-Crofts, 1967

Potasznik H, Nelson G: Stress and social support: the burden experienced
by the family of the mentally ill person. Am J Community Psychiatry
12:509–607, 1984

Rabkin J: Public attitudes toward mental illness: a review of the literature.
Schizophr Bull 10:9–33, 1974

Reynolds I, Hoult JE: The relatives of the mentally ill: a comparative trial of
community-oriented psychiatric care. J Nerv Ment Dis 172:480–489, 1984

Rice EP, Ekdahl MC, Miller L: Children of Mentally Ill Parents: Problems in
Child Care. New York, Behavioral Publications, 1971

Rogler LH, Hollingshead AR: Trapped: Families and Schizophrenia. New
York, John Wiley, 1965

Runck B: The mentally ill at home: a family matter, in Families Today: A
Research Sampler on Families and Children, Vol 2 (DHEW Publ No
(ADM) 79-898). Edited by Corfman E. Washington, DC, U.S. Govern-
ment Printing Office, 1979

Sameroff AJ, Zax M: In search of schizophrenia: young offspring of schizophrenic women, in The Nature of Schizophrenia. Edited by Wynne L,
Cromwell R, Matthyse S. New York, John Wiley, 1978

Schulz PM, Schulz SC, Targum SD, et al: Patient and family attitudes about
schizophrenia: implications for genetic counseling. Schizophr Bull 8:504–
513, 1982

Smets AC: Family and staff attitudes toward family involvement in the treatment of hospitalized chronic patients. Hosp Community Psychiatry 33:573–
575, 1982

Smith CM: Measuring some effects of mental illness on the home. Canadian
Psychiatric Association Journal 14:97–104, 1969

Spaniol L, Jung H, Zipple AM, et al: Families as a central resource in the
rehabilitation of the severely psychiatrically disabled: report of a national
survey. Unpublished manuscript, Boston University, Center for Rehabilitation Research and Training in Mental Health, 1984

Spitzer SP, Weinstein RM, Nelson ML: Family reaction and career of the psychiatric patient: a long-term follow-up study, in The Psychiatric Hospital and the Family. Edited by Harbin HT. New York, SP Medical & Scientific Books, 1982, pp 187–212

Stein LI, Test MA: Alternatives to mental hospital treatment: conceptual model, treatment program, and clinical evaluation. Arch Gen Psychiatry 37:392–399, 1980

Stratton JM, Seman PM: Family therapy supervision on a psychiatric inpatient unit: implications of an ecological epistemology, in The Psychiatric Hospital and the Family. Edited by Harbin T. New York, SP Medical & Scientific Books, 1982, pp 309–334

Tarrier N, Barrowclough C, Vaughn C, et al: The community management of schizophrenia: a controlled trial of a behavioural intervention with families to reduce relapse. Br J Psychiatry 153:532–542, 1988

Terkelsen KG: Schizophrenia and the family: adverse effects of family therapy. Fam Proc 22:191–200, 1983

Test MA, Stein LI: Alternatives to mental hospital treatment, IV: social cost. Arch Gen Psychiatry 37:409–412, 1980

Thompson EH, Doll W: The burden of families coping with the mentally ill: an invisible crisis. Family Relations 31:379–388, 1982

Vaughn CE, Leff JP: The influence of family and social factors on the course of psychiatric illness. Br J Psychiatry 129:125–137, 1976

Vine P: Families in Pain: Children, Siblings, Spouses, and Parents Speak Out. New York, Pantheon, 1982

Weinstein SE: The family of the chronic mental patient: ally or adversary? in The Psychiatric Hospital and the Family. Edited by Harbin HT. New York, SP Medical & Scientific Books, 1982, pp 297–308

Wender PH, Rosenthal D, Zahn TP, et al: The psychiatric adjustment of the adopting parents of schizophrenics. Am J Psychiatry 122:1013–1018, 1971

Wynne L, Singer MT: Thought disorder and family relations of schizophrenics, I: a research strategy. Arch Gen Psychiatry 9:191–198, 1963

Commentary to Chapter 2

Can the Family Literature Be Integrated?

William R. McFarlane, M.D.

Dr. Johnson has done an admirable service for all who are concerned with the families of the mentally ill. In his review, we see reflected from the literature an image of the complex and stressful difficulties faced and endured by family members, usually alone, attempting to cope with the prolonged agonies of schizophrenia and other major psychiatric disorders. It is a disheartening image in the sense that it provokes a deeper appreciation for what families have lacked from professionals—empathy, workable guidance, emotional support, and respite; in short, the right attitude. His chapter and many of the cited references should be required reading for all professionals who work with the mentally ill and their families.

In one sense, a discussion of the chapter could stop there. What this commentary addresses is the emergence of a dichotomous family literature, which in turn describes a dichotomous family and which arises from a potentially dichotomized professional community. The problem is this: The family is portrayed either as burdened by or as a negative influence on the mentally ill family member, but rarely as both and rarely as a major resource in treatment. Dr. Johnson has ameliorated this problem by going beyond the burden literature and emphasizing the positive influences families have on their ill relatives and the contributory role they can play given the necessary resources and supports. What I would like to do by way of discussion is to outline this dichotomy as a serious problem and to propose a framework within which to think about a solution.

Perhaps one way to introduce the problem of this dichotomous family literature is to share a few salient details of my own professional education. During rotations on psychiatry and neurology in medical school, I was taught consistently that there were no anatomical, biochemical, physiological, or histopathological abnormalities in the brains of patients with schizophrenia. Only Franz Kallman's twin studies suggested that there might be a biological component in the development of the illness. On the other hand, there was considerable time devoted to teaching about the psychodynamics of psychosis, and some attention, largely critical, was given to the role of parents in fostering and reinforcing their ill child's flight from reality.

During my residency, these themes were elaborated further, especially in the seemingly elegant construct of the double-bind hypothesis, in the observations of the schismatic and skewed marriages of the patient's parents, in the three-generational transmission theory, and so on. This education led to seeing the family as a problem but also as a possible source of help for the patient, because on closer inspection many families did not seem to have such negative effects on the patient. Through all of it there lingered the nagging question of why the phenothiazines seemed to be so effective in reducing or even eliminating psychotic symptoms, independent of family or other social influences. My formal professional education ended with this question unanswered.

The only real help came later from Albert Scheflen (1981), to whom we are indebted for pointing the way to a multilevel construct. He reinforced the notion that biological and psychophysiological factors must play a role in the etiology of the disorder and that much of what looked like family dysfunction could well be secondary, i.e., the family attempting to deal with a major and mystifying illness. Further, he insisted on using systems thinking in its basic scientific sense; for instance, he proposed that positive feedback loops in a family would involve reciprocal effects between an illness in one member and everyone else, leading to a gradual deterioration in the functioning and well-being of all concerned. We will return to this crucial notion later.

The problem of a bipartite family literature can be seen as another sign of an emerging overemphasis on a one-factor causal model, which Scheflen (1981), Spring and Zubin (1978), and others have urged to abandon. In its essence, our problem is the lack of integration of the increasingly abundant and sophisticated evidence for devastating burdens on the well members of the family with the similarly reliable evidence that those same members have powerful positive and negative effects on their ill relative. In the literature, the family has been sundered into two nearly adversarial camps: the patient versus everyone else. Of course, there is some basis for such a dichotomy—usually only one member of a given family has a major psychiatric disorder. The well members and the ill member have very different experiences and are usefully separated for purposes of research analysis.

However, the emerging problem, which is more disturbing and must soon be addressed by educators of professionals, is that there has been a tendency to leave this dichotomy intact. It appears that the professional community is at risk of reifying this division by allowing itself to be defined by which part of the family it supports. Further, there is the specter that those who attempt to *fully* understand family effects on the patient will be seen as continuing uncritically the now discredited tradition of casually blaming the family for the illness, for want of a better explanation. Likewise, the burden literature and those who work in that area could be seen as the only truly profamily wing of the field. An exaggeration of this division is problematic for at least three reasons: 1) it could potentially impede scientific and clinical advances; 2) it would exaggerate the confusion, anger, and demoralization felt by many families about the negative-influence literature; and 3) it would leave educators and supervisors in a paralyzing dilemma. That is, how is one to teach trainees about both sets of studies, or should one even try? For instance, by teaching trainees about expressed emotion and communication deviance is one risking fostering in them a blaming ideological construct, one that is likely to have adverse effects on families? Is a thorough familiarity with the burden literature a sufficient safeguard against such an outcome? Could it, on the other hand, leave clinicians helpless to offer guidance about preferable interactional styles when that is indicated?

What follows is a set of propositions that might be of assistance in moving us beyond this dichotomy. By way of acknowledgment, we should note that Anderson et al. (1986) have done much to foster the kind of integration that I am urging here, as have Scheflen (1981) and Beels (see commentary to Chapter 7, this volume). If we were to reach a consensus based on any one of their views, we would have advanced far already.

VARIATION AMONG FAMILIES

The first integrating proposition is that families of the mentally ill vary enormously, something inadequately taken into account in either body of literature. They are best seen within an epidemiologic perspective, as a population with normal variation on any kind of global measure of functional adaptiveness and on many, if not all, measures of structure, interaction, experience, and performance.

For example, Miklowitz et al. (1986) recently found that communication deviance (CD), often cited as a nearly universal characteristic of families with a schizophrenic member, actually is clustered among relatives who are also overinvolved; low expressed emotion (EE) and critical relatives were statistically indistinguishable in their levels of CD, which were significantly lower. The low-EE group, in fact, was all but lacking CD. The overinvolved high-CD subgroup represented only 16% of the total sample. Also, there were significant differences between relative subgroups—fathers were generally lower than mothers or other key relatives on the sum EE score, whereas mothers were more overinvolved and fathers more critical. Sturgeon et al. (1981) and Tarrier et al. (1979) found that the presence of high-EE relatives was associated with increased arousal and instability in their schizophrenic family member, whereas the presence of a low-EE relative appeared to produce not only decreased arousal, but also rapid accommodation to an unfamiliar interviewer. Such accommodation generally is rare in schizophrenic patients, suggesting that some family members induce unusually positive therapeutic effects.

In a more impressionistic vein, as we have recruited and worked closely with a large sample of patients with schizophrenia and their families at six hospitals distributed across New York State, we have been amazed and at times overwhelmed by the variety of styles, strengths, and weaknesses of these families. The same kind of variation characterizes their experience of the illness. Despite some similarities of the degree and type of objective burden, family members do not all respond in similar ways. Some actually appear to be immune to extreme distress, a factor we believe portends well for the patient.

The observations that relatives with a low-EE style have a noticeably salutary effect on relapse frequency, accommodation to strangers, and social/vocational adjustment of their mentally ill family members depend on an assumption of wide variation between families. They have had great clinical significance by pointing to the potential value of the psychoeducational approaches. We made the same assumption in our recent study, in which we have found an association between mothers' emotional overinvolvement and their prior experience of being stigmatized and rejected themselves—as the relative of a mentally ill individual—but only when their social networks are adequate. Put simply, some relatives are stigmatized, some are overinvolved, and many are both, but most are neither. Clinically, this finding suggests that multifamily and self-help groups might counteract tendencies toward overinvolvement by reducing stigma, when it is present.

To summarize, this view implies that a few families are especially healthy, some are particularly dysfunctional, and the rest are in-between, and thereby ordinary. It is clear that clinicians need to take that variation into account in deciding how to help a given family cope with a mental illness in their midst.

Specifically, given the findings from recent and more rigorous studies, it seems all but meaningless to speak of "the family," let alone a schizophrenogenic family, if only because it now seems clear that many relatives seem capable of *enhancing* the compensation and re-habilitation of their ill family members. As did Bleuler (1911) with regard to schizophrenia itself, we should accept this variety as a given, and as one way to account for many seemingly contradictory findings and as a guide to refining clinical strategies.

The second proposition follows from the first. A useful point of departure for developing an integrated view of the family is that family variation should be viewed as orthogonal to variation in the illness; if you will, a macro–null hypothesis. Then, the relationship of family functioning to onset or subsequent course should be inves-tigated empirically, and not assumed. This view obligates us to look at, for instance, whether aspects of family burden are associated with poor clinical outcome, as well as with more fully investigated factors like EE.

A most intriguing example of following this general direction is another Miklowitz (1983) study in which emotional overinvolvement was found to be associated with poor premorbid adjustment. Thereby, he may have helped us understand a source of overinvolvement: one interpretation of this finding is that overinvolvement might result from the relative's concern about, and need to compensate for, pre-morbid disability in the schizophrenic-to-be. It is a short step to seeing overinvolvement as a natural, perhaps adaptive, reaction to the bur-den of attempting to cope with a subtly and mysteriously impaired child. In our present research studies, we are pursuing a similar path, trying to understand the relationship of differences in degree and type of experienced burden and stigma to course of illness and to EE.

FEEDBACK CONCEPT

The third proposition is that, at least for heuristic purposes, we begin to define relationships linking family experience, family inter-action, and course of illness as feedback loops rather than as seemingly simpler causal relationships. A principal reason to do so is that the major disorders have such long-term courses that it is nearly incon-ceivable that there are not reciprocal and sequential effects of illness on family and family on illness. Such a conceptual framework seems to make the integration of the reliable "burden" and "negative influ-ence" studies more feasible by linking them in a reciprocal interaction hypothesis. A suggestion of this kind of factor interaction is found in Vaughn and Leff's (1976) content analysis of the comments of high-

EE relatives in their London sample: The family members, in essence, were angry about negative symptoms. To many of us, that represents an effect of the lack of education, a lack that appears as an aspect of subjective burden in many of the self-report studies reviewed by Johnson. Falloon and Pederson (1985) have shown that a family management approach that provides education and guidance reduces EE, relapse frequency, and severity of perceived burden, while improving coping skills. This finding fits a feedback model involving all four factors.

It seems reasonable, for example, to construct a positive feedback hypothesis in which negative symptoms beget in relatives exasperation and anger, which are expressed increasingly as critical comments, which lead to clinical deterioration, which begets more family exasperation, and so on, spiraling progressively through time, at least until relapse temporarily breaks the cycle. Although such a concept does a better job of reflecting a very complex reality, it renders linear causal relationships between any two factors less explanatory and less useful. It also, I believe, makes it possible for clinicians to have a deeper understanding of the predicament of all family members simultaneously, patient included, without having to take sides. At the conceptual level, it leaves the family intact, with schizophrenia as a chronic disorder being the principal concern of patient, relatives, and clinician alike.

A corollary of the feedback concept is that burden and negative family influences can be generated from outside the family boundary, especially through the way the immediate family's network and community respond to the illness. I have mentioned our finding that social network and stigma interact powerfully with mothers' overinvolvement with patients, suggesting that extrafamily social influences may contribute to a clinical outcome. Further, the strongest correlation with overinvolvement in that study has been with cramped housing, suggesting that the sources of overinvolvement might include more mundane factors like available space, cultural styles, and family economics. There is abundant evidence in Johnson's review that the way the clinical staff (an extrafamily influence) responds to families can and does induce guilt, anger, and demoralization, which are most likely to lead to less-than-ideal responses by family members to symptoms and disability in the patient. Regardless of any existing findings, we could well propose that research that investigates negative family influences ultimately should be as concerned with their sources as their effects. It seems realistic to assume that, if we can understand the latter, we can understand the former. We may need to look to the family's context for positive answers.

ENVIRONMENTAL INFLUENCES

The fourth proposition is that family experience and especially negative family influences should be seen as only one subset of a larger category: environmental influences in general. This notion relates directly to schizophrenia, but may apply to affective disorders and the severe personality disorders as well. Schizophrenia is, if nothing else, a vulnerability to becoming cognitively disorganized under the influence of environmental factors that produce stimulus overload, especially social ambiguity and excessive complexity, social intrusiveness, strong or negative emotions, pressure to perform and compete, sexual stimulation, and excessive noise. Family life in modern America is rife with all of these factors, nearly as the norm to be lived up to. But so is urban life generally and so is life in the average psychiatric inpatient unit and day hospital. Though lacking rigor, it is meaningful to speak of high EE as the family version of negative intensity found in all kinds of social environments. Studies by Linn et al. (1979, 1980) of day hospitals and foster homes strongly suggest that inappropriate expectations, high levels of social stimulation, emphasis on internal experience, and lack of structure yield poor outcome when coming from professionals and nonkin caretakers. Put another way, if we have learned that family members make mistakes in dealing with their ill relative and that those mistakes do indeed lead to a poor clinical outcome, then we should also have learned that clinicians and the lay public make all the same mistakes and contribute equally to the misery of the person with schizophrenia. The common denominator is a lack of appreciation for the schizophrenic person's profound inability to regulate arousal and process information. For instance, is not social rejection based on stigma a society-wide version of critical comments, delivered in some instances nonverbally? Is the demand that patients immediately enter occupational training programs the day after discharge from a brief inpatient stay, often while still residually psychotic, an example of overly ambitious expectations? Shouldn't we be concerned that intensive psychodynamic psychotherapy of schizophrenia may be a form of overinvolvement?

It might help to integrate families and clinicians, as well as the respective literatures, if we see some of the driving forces behind all these negative factors as similar. Certainly, most serious clinicians dealing with schizophrenia have experienced the exasperation, anger, confusion, mystification, and demoralization that families describe (and that probably play a part in high EE). Committed clinicians know what burden is, at least in an attenuated form. At the core of both the relative's and the clinician's problems is the same factor: ignorance about what to do, about what is helpful. It is only very recently that we have been clear empirically about what drives the schizophrenic patient into, and what seems to be protective against, relapse. One can read the research as suggesting that we are all—family and clinicians alike—pushing patients too much, expecting too much, and trying too hard to make them better. This is certainly one interpretation of the Veterans Administration day hospital and foster home studies by Linn et al. (1979, 1980). In other words, less is in many ways better. Of course, that principle is one of the core elements of the psychoeducational family programs, which improve clinical outcome, reduce family burden, and prevent exhaustion. Perhaps it goes without saying, but is also clear, that burdens experienced by relatives are greater and more persistent than any comparable experiences of clinicians or the general public.

CONTINUITY OF CARE

This last difference leads to the fifth and final proposition: we must appreciate and teach that, even if family members have negative effects on their ill relative, they do one thing that compensates mightily: they care deeply and they do so for the long haul. Continuity of care is debated and often advocated in clinical circles; in families it is a given. The clinical effects of this caring are evident in several studies: Steinberg and Durell (1968) documented what everyone knows—that the illness begins in nearly every instance when the victim leaves home to try to become an autonomous adult, that is, gets out of range of family support. Mosher's Soteria House (Mosher et al. 1975), Fairweather's lodges (1980), and Stein and Test's community treatment program (1978) illustrate how well things turn out when the treatment tries to be as pervasively supportive, empathic, and committed as the most ordinary of families are as a matter of course. Family members will almost always be more positive and feel more affection than clinicians, because they knew the patient before he or she became ill and because blood is still far thicker than water. These affectional bonds should be of interest to other than budgeteers looking for less expensive alternatives to supervised residences. For clinicians, they are an essential element in a successful treatment plan and therefore need and should receive protection, reinforcement, validation, and emulation. I concur with Dr. Johnson in urging that we cease immediately writing and speaking of family members in anything like pejorative terms. Instead, we must address them as respected collaborators and colleagues, who can with support and guidance provide what the mentally ill need and are unlikely to receive from clinicians—permanent and loving commitment.

SUMMARY

By way of summary, it may suffice to urge that the education of professionals should be nothing less than comprehensive and inclusive. If clinical and research trainees are encouraged to read and think about all of the better research on families, they would be likely to arrive at conclusions similar to the propositions suggested here. On the other hand, if we continue the trend to define all families as alike and to emphasize only negative effects on well family members of the ill member or only negative effects of well family members on the ill member, we run a real danger of turning out either confused or inappropriately partisan clinicians who will surely be less than useful to families and patients, regardless of which side they take. The same argument applies to research and researchers.

In that regard, it is of some concern that some family advocates have seen investigation of family effects on schizophrenia as necessarily blaming families in general. Were it not for earlier studies of this type, we might not have today those psychoeducational family programs that seem to meet many of the stated needs of family members. We need to understand the contextual or inherited sources of high EE and CD to help families put these factors in the perspective they deserve—that is, that they are extremely unlikely to be unilaterally causal and could as well be secondary as primary, based on present knowledge. We need to know more about low EE and "emotional expressiveness," as termed in Spiegel and Wissler's recent study (1986), because we still have much to learn about the optional social environment for schizophrenia, at various phases. Families have much to teach in this regard. Relatives and clinicians need to accept that patients with schizophrenia require a special social environment to reach their full potential; anyone can affect the ill person, all too easily, because of the peculiar vulnerabilities produced by the disorder. That one has a major effect on the patient is, therefore, not a measure of good or bad parenting or clinical practice, but of schizophrenia itself.

To go one step further, we need to know if family interaction or nonkin contextual factors are contributory to the onset of the manifest illness, because we are close to knowing enough to identify children at biological risk for schizophrenia. Their families, if given well-designed specific guidance, would become essential collaborators in any effort to prevent the initial episode. If this kind of secondary prevention proved feasible, it would be worth the temporary embarrassment to the family of being asked to adopt new, somewhat abnormal modes of compensatory interaction with the vulnerable child. Ultimately, one way of reducing family burden in schizophrenia is to try to reduce the frequency and severity of psychotic episodes to the absolute minimum.

The family—here I mean the entire family, including the patient—is one of the prime vehicles for achieving that goal. The other side of the coin is that clinicians need to pay close attention to what family research is telling us about negative social factors, so that we start to alter our interactions with patients in ways similar to those being suggested for relatives. Further, professionals clearly need to alter their behavior with relatives in ways suggested by the self-report studies reviewed by Dr. Johnson. If all these improvements begin to happen on a wide scale, the prognosis for the entire family—well members and ill—will greatly improve.

REFERENCES

Anderson CM, Reiss DJ, Hogarty GE: Schizophrenia and the Family. New York, Guilford, 1986

Bleuler E: Dementia Praecox, or the Group of Schizophrenias (1911). Translated by Zinkin J. New York, International Universities Press, 1950

Falloon IRH, Pederson J: Family management in the prevention of morbidity of schizophrenia: the adjustment of the family unit. Br J Psychiatry 147:156–163, 1985

Fairweather GW: The Fairweather Lodge: a twenty-five year retrospective. New Dir Ment Health Serv 7:1–13, 1980

Linn NW, Caffey EM, Klett CJ, et al: Day treatment and psychotropic drugs in the aftercare of schizophrenic patients. Arch Gen Psychiatry 36:1055–1066, 1979

Linn NW, Klett CJ, Caffey EM: Foster home characteristics and psychiatric patient outcome. Arch Gen Psychiatry 37:129–132, 1980

Miklowitz DJ, Goldstein MJ, Falloon IRH: Premorbid and symptomatic characteristics of schizophrenics from families with high and low levels of expressed emotion. J Abnorm Psychol 92:359–367, 1983

Miklowitz DJ, Strachan AM, Goldstein MJ, et al: Expressed emotion and communication deviance in the families of schizophrenics. J Abnorm Psychol 95:60–66, 1986

Mosher LR, Menn A, Matthews SM: Soteria: evaluation of a home-based treatment for schizophrenia. Am J Orthopsychiatry 45:455–467, 1975

Scheflen A: Levels of Schizophrenia. New York, Brunner/Mazel, 1981

Spiegel D, Wissler T: Family environment as a predictor of psychiatric rehospitalization. Am J Psychiatry 143:56–60, 1986

Spring BJ, Zubin J: Attention and information processing as indicators of vulnerability to schizophrenic episodes, in The Nature of Schizophrenia. Edited by Wynne LC, Cromwell RL, Matthyse S. New York, John Wiley, 1978

Stein LI, Test MA (eds): Alternatives to Mental Hospital Treatment. New York, Plenum, 1978

Steinberg HR, Durell JA: A stressful social situation as a precipitant of schizophrenia. Br J Psychiatry 114:1097–1105, 1968

Sturgeon D, Kuipers L, Berkowitz R, et al: Psychophysiological responses of schizophrenic patients to high and low expressed emotion relatives. Br J Psychiatry 138:40–45, 1981

Tarrier N, Vaughn CE, Lader MH, et al: Bodily responses to people and events in schizophrenics. Arch Gen Psychiatry 36:311–315, 1979

Vaughn CE, Leff JP: The influence of family and social factors on the course of psychiatric illness. Br J Psychiatry 129:125–137, 1976

Chapter 3

The Social Context of Helping Families

Agnes B. Hatfield, Ph.D.

Difficulties in solving human problems arise, in part, because they are viewed in isolation from the larger social context in which they are embedded. Programs of social service fail to successfully remediate these problems when they ignore the social framework of which they are a part. The political, social, and historical contexts of the time too often go unnoticed and unexamined (Bachrach 1987; Hersch 1972; Levine 1981; Sarason 1981). Faced with a dilemma, as we are, as to how to help families cope with mental illness, we cannot afford to disregard the wider context in which the problem is embedded.

No social reform takes place in isolation. The condition and spirit of the time and its social, political, and economic characteristics strongly influence the problems that concern us, the principles and theories that we use to guide us, and the helping forms that are developed (Hersch 1972). We must, then, guard against the common tendency to assume that it is possible to think and act independently of the forces around us.

Sarason (1981) identified psychologists as a professional group who have "never been able to confront directly that the substance of their theories cannot be independent of who and where psychologists are in the society in which they have been socialized" (p. 15). However, the same criticism can probably be leveled at all mental health disciplines. One of the sources of difficulty, Sarason informed us, is the inability to fathom that every person has a worldview that provides the context for ordering life, which encompasses his or her past, present, and future. No one views others or the world around them from a completely objective point of view. "We are inevitably prisoners of time, place, and culture" noted Sarason (p. 47), and even more to the point, he reminded us that "one's worldview of the universe is interwoven with one's view of people" (p. 46). Sarason's point of view is essential in helping us understand why there is such a great diversity in the theory and practice of family intervention. No theorist or practitioner comes to the field with a purely objective point of view; each is necessarily a product of personal history and the historical period in which he or she lives. Our purpose in this book is to arrive at the system of help for families most appropriate to families in the present social context.

It is useful to recognize, however, that identifying or creating the most appropriate modality of help is not the end of the matter, for change does not necessarily come about in a planned and coordinated way. There are many social factors that influence change, and the more these are identified and understood at the outset, the more likely it is that plans can be brought to fruition. There is, of course, great separation and dispersion of powers between various levels of government and between the public and private sectors. Some, said Levine (1981), have the power to order and influence others; others have the power to resist or redirect resources. Family advocates have come to understand the need to thoroughly understand the political games that are played. Politics are not wrong and are bad only if we blind ourselves to their inevitability (Levine 1981). Even more, as Rochefort (1984) wrote, "We ought to consider not only the state of present policy, but also the state of the iceberg of dynamic social perceptions and attitudes that underlies it" (p. 26). While we need to keep this worthy objective before us, we will necessarily have to settle for more modest goals. We have chosen to discuss four social forces that we believe must be understood as we plan programs of help to families: our concept of rights and responsibilities, tradition and nature of professional help giving, the family consumer advocacy movement, and the trend toward fiscal restraint.

CONCEPT OF RIGHTS AND RESPONSIBILITIES

A body of literature now exists that clearly demonstrates that managing a highly disturbed psychiatrically disabled adult in the home can be one of the most overwhelming experiences that a family may ever undergo (Hatfield 1978; Hatfield and Lefley 1987; Holden and Lewine 1982; Lefley 1987; Potasznik and Nelson 1984). Moreover, legal developments in the past two decades have made the problem still more complicated. Under the doctrine of "least restrictive environment" based on an interpretation of the First Amendment of the Constitution, even the most severely disturbed persons cannot be involuntarily held in hospitals in most states unless they are clearly dangerous to self or others. To a family whose relative is obviously decompensating, highly delusional, neglecting minimal health and safety standards, and desperately in need of treatment, the present state is incomprehensible. They have difficulty believing that a sane society expects a highly disordered brain to make rational decisions about the need for treatment or that caring families must stand by and wait until something dangerous happens and treatment can be compelled. Nevertheless, this is the strange dilemma of our time. Klein (1983), formerly with the Mental Health Law Project, now believes that the doctrine of least restrictive environment is fundamentally flawed. Treatment and liberty, he asserts, cannot be treated as independent variables. It places least restrictiveness as a higher value than safety and efficacy. Klein believes we may be at a watershed on this issue and that courts may soon restore civil commitment to a meaningful form of intervention aimed at providing treatment. Because families are so intimately affected by the options they have when dealing with a very disturbed relative, how this issue of involuntary treatment plays itself out in the next few years will be a significant factor in conceptualizing the help that families will need.

The question of who is legally responsible for the care of psychiatrically disabled adults in this country is another thorny issue that baffles families. The resolution of that issue also affects the help that families need. In the early days of deinstitutionalization, families assumed that the public was responsible and could be compelled to provide food, shelter, and treatment for disabled adults. However, Klein (1983) said, "Regrettably, there is no general legal right to services in our society. A legal right, as distinguished from a moral or ethical right, is one that is enforceable in court. There is no right to good housing. There is no right to adequate food. Indeed, despite many legal challenges in the later 1960s, it now appears generally accepted that there is no right for any largesse provided by our Constitution" (p. 108).

Who then is accountable for seeing that the psychiatrically disabled survive in the community? In most states, relatives (other than spouses) are not legally responsible for the care of a psychiatrically disabled adult. Presumably, as long as he or she is not involuntarily held someplace, the mentally ill person is legally responsible for his or her own care. However, people with severe disorders cannot take this responsibility, and their survival depends on the moral and ethical commitment of others in the society. Most frequently it is the family, then, that feels morally bound to ensure its relative's well-being. For the time being, families have been willing to provide direct care in the family home, but the evidence is that they do not consider this a

long-term solution. Although there may not be constitutional entitlements to care in the community, there are statutes providing for
housing, food, and general welfare, and these can be augmented,
given strong advocacy, so that persons with mental illnesses can live
independent of their immediate relatives.

There is a growing fear among members of the National Alliance
for the Mentally Ill (NAMI), the rapidly growing consumer advocacy
movement in this country, that significant investment in the training
of professionals in family education and treatment will result in a de
facto decision that families should be care givers. There is fear that
this might occur without any kind of high-level discussion in which
families themselves are involved. If a large cadre of professionals are
trained to give therapy or psychoeducational interventions to the family, would not their own self-interest, then, lead them to advocate that
these families (with treatment, of course) be assigned the direct care-
giving role (Hatfield et al. 1987)?

Almost certainly, the decision as to who provides direct care will
be resolved politically. Given NAMI's increasing political clout, it is
important to note that advocacy on the state level is directed first and
foremost to housing. None of the replies to a recent NAMI question-
naire indicated that families were advocating treatment for themselves. Families clearly believe that tax dollars are better invested in
training first-rate staff and providing residences than are dollars invested in parenting. This seems to contradict earlier findings (Hatfield
1979; Holden and Lewine 1982) that families do feel the need for
professional help. What we believe families are saying is that they
want to understand mental illness, they may need support in their
grief and disappointment, and they want guidance in establishing
limited but more meaningful contacts with their disturbed relative.
This help should be short-term, nonintrusive, and directed at the
specific concerns families identify. It should be low in cost so as not
to divert too many dollars from the more important goal of community care for the mentally ill person.

Tradition and Nature of
Professional Help Giving

In our culture, when mental illness strikes a member, families
naturally turn to the mental health profession to seek treatment for
the patient and advice for themselves. This is a fairly typical medical
model; it is what a family would do if its relative had pneumonia,
diabetes, or any other serious ailment. What families find, however,
is the response to them as families is very different from that experienced with other medical specialties. It is the purpose of this section

to explore some of the aspects of the mental health subculture that have been problematic to families.

One of the first things that families may discover on seeking help is the prevailing ideology that anyone who seeks help is by definition "sick." Pathology, it seems, is everywhere. Mental health professionals have tended to ignore the objective fact of stressful environments that might, indeed, overwhelm the strongest of us. Whether the problems are existential, ethical, or political, professionals behave as though a therapeutic philosophy or method can cure (Gartner and Riessman 1977).

Psychiatry, said Penfold and Walker (1983), has "power over the very way in which our lives are made sensible, made rational, made comprehensible." This, they said, is what we mean by "ideology." Ideology provides an explanation that obscures actuality and that legitimates the position of those who create it. Psychiatry and its allied disciplines have the power to define what is normal and to insist that their definition must be valid for the rest of us (Penfold and Walker 1983; Morris 1978).

It was this therapeutic climate that families stumbled into in their often nearly desperate search for practical assistance in dealing with a severely disturbed family member. Although by any objective standard these families were faced with problems in the environment of severe proportions, the mental health professional redefined the problem as one of family deficit, dysfunction, or pathology and offered them the curative powers of therapy. This added to the family's shame and anxiety, but many, out of a desperate need to do anything humanly possible to help their relative, subjected themselves to some form of therapy. Others scoffed at the irrationality of the idea that they were the sick ones and became alienated from the mental health profession.

The emphasis in the professions on the normal and the abnormal turned out on closer examination to be labels for good and bad behavior. This is a source of great suffering for those so labeled. Families of the mentally ill were not the first to rebel against such designations. It is instructive to note how other stigmatized groups reacted to it.

For many years, homosexuals suffered ridicule and ostracism at the hands of those who knew of their deviance. They finally rose up and formed a militant social action group whose mission was to oppose society's negative stereotype. The Gay Liberation Front, as the group was called, was particularly incensed by psychiatry's definition of its members' sexual preferences as evidence of pathology. In the words of Bayer (1981), the Gay Liberation Front "in a mood of militancy rose up to challenge what they considered the unwarranted, burdensome, and humiliating domination of psychiatry. Armed with the techniques of social protest, they subjected American psychiatry to a series of jolts" (p. 9). Responding to destructive techniques at meetings of the American Psychiatric Association (APA) and after several years of bitter dispute, APA decided to remove homosexuality from the *Diagnostic and Statistical Manual of Mental Disorders*, its official list of mental diseases. Infuriated by this decision, dissident psychiatrists asked that the issue be submitted to a referendum of its members. Thus, members voted on what was once considered a scientific question. Such a dramatic removal raises the question of how a pattern of sexual behavior can be classified as pathological one day and not the next, noted Bayer in his summary of this unusual event.

Other groups have also used the techniques of social protest to achieve change in the way they are defined by mental health professionals. Women have criticized the professions for their patriarchal, autocratic, and coercive techniques and values (Chesler 1972; Penfold and Walker 1983). By assuming an air of omniscience and benevolent superiority, psychiatrists, they feel, foster submission, dependency, and infantilism, which reinforces the stereotype of what the typical woman is like. Women's perspectives have been unrepresented or underrepresented in American psychiatric journals and textbooks. The woman's point of view—the female experience—has traditionally been stated by male psychiatrists. Change did not come about by the discovery of new theory or launching of new research; it came about because of political necessity.

Until a decade or so ago, the family experience with mental illness was invariably described by the mental health professional performing the treatment and rarely by the persons undergoing the experience. It is only in recent years as families have gained a voice that we have learned how invalid and damaging some of these perceptions and problem definitions really were. It might be apt, in relation to this issue, to present briefly the plight of another group of beleaguered families who felt blamed and rejected as they struggled with one of life's most painful tragedies—the families of autistic children. Autism was first identified by psychiatric professionals; thus, it was defined as a psychiatric illness, and families, especially mothers, were blamed for causing it. Intensive psychodynamic approaches did nothing to solve the problems. Ritvo (1976) credits Fenichel with advocating a break with the traditional doctrine, and he credits Rimland with the intensive effort to get rid of the "noxious parent" label. The National Society for Autistic Children takes the position that autism is not an emotional disorder and that its treatment does not lie in the realm of mental health, but rather that autism is a neurological disorder and its victims can best be helped through education. The parallel between the evolution of thinking about autism and that of the major mental illnesses is not lost on families of patients with these latter disorders.

Confidence in the mental health profession is diminished by the excessive diversity within the field about how to help families. A common topic in family support groups is the many kinds of contradictory advice they receive about the same kinds of problems. The consumer does not know whom to believe. A sampling of leading mental health journals in the last couple of years would surely find professionals with their theoretical investments in psychoanalysis, behaviorism, cognitive psychology, and a great diversity of family theories. Their assumptions about mental illness and its etiology are tied to almost every possible style of family interaction, family pattern and organization, and communication style. Contradictions between professional ideas abound, thus diminishing credibility in the eyes of the public. What is needed is reform from within the professions. Surely no professional finds each of these diverse beliefs equally defensible; yet the whole profession is tarnished by some of the weird ideas and practices of members. Mental health professionals are not social reformers within their professional group. They aren't whistle blowers—they believe in live and let live. "It is not scandalous conditions that are troublesome," Levine (1981) insisted, "it is scandal."

The social critic Ivan Illich (1977) notes a progressive alienation of the world of ordinary men and women from the elites who rule in the name of superior and inaccessible knowledge. They mask their autocratic acts, Illich (1975) insists, with a benign ideology of service. Bayer (1981) feels Illich's point of view is representative of a significant and growing segment of the population. This is harsh criticism that may apply just as well to other businesses and professions that have something to sell to the public. The tendency, however, is to react with greater cynicism, because we have been deluded, or have chosen to delude ourselves, into thinking that providing mental health services is a wholly selfless endeavor.

The social context in which professionals work influences and constrains what they can do. Users of services must understand these realities and make their decisions accordingly. Providers of service are organized into professional groups, and it is their activities and the political issues behind them that give shape to service delivery. Services to those in need are mediated by agencies and professionals who have their own vital concerns. In theory, mental health professionals approach the task of improving services in the light of what contemporary knowledge and theory says is best (Harshbarger 1978; Levine 1981). However, behind the mask of the desire to help people, McKnight (1977) reminds us, are services, their systems, techniques, and technologies—businesses in need of markets, an economy seeking new growth potential, professionals in need of an income. All are legitimate concerns, but consumers must know these realities and not delude themselves into thinking that all clinical decisions are made on the basis of love and care. Clinicians, McKnight says, do manufacture needs in order to have something to treat. Professionals need to see people in terms of personal deficiency.

The Zeitgeist of our time is one in which the early post–World War II optimism about mental health service has soured considerably (Levine 1981). Whether the field can and will change in time to hold onto families of the mentally ill as clientele is a question. Clinicians might turn on themselves the techniques they use to pry into their clients' motives, values, and needs to understand themselves. Clinicians are, of course, entitled to their needs and values, but when fulfilling the needs of the clinician is disabling to families, then families must go elsewhere for help.

FAMILY CONSUMER ADVOCACY MOVEMENT

Any discussion of the social context of mental health service provision must necessarily give due attention to the rapid growth of consumer advocacy organizations in this country, of which NAMI is probably the best example in the field of mental health. At its first organizing meeting in 1979, then director of the National Institute of Mental Health Dr. Herbert Pardes stated in a major address to participants that the development of NAMI might well be the most important influence in mental health in a decade (National Alliance for the Mentally Ill 1979). Torrey (1983) made an even stronger prediction in which he saw the growth of NAMI as "the single biggest advance in coping with schizophrenia since the introduction of antipsychotic drugs" (p. 179).

Because consumer movements are also embedded in a social context and they are products of a time and a place, it is instructive to consider factors that gave rise to these developments—both to understand the movement as such and to understand some of the wider forces affecting mental health provision generally. NAMI had its origins in 1) deinstitutionalization and the return of mentally ill persons to the community to live, 2) the large percentage of families involved in direct care giving, 3) disenchantment with mental health professionals who lacked sympathy for the problems of care giving and failed to provide the practical help needed, 4) tendencies of professionals to blame families for their relative's mental illness or to see families in pejorative ways, and 5) lack of community resources to maximize patient rehabilitation. In addition to these various negative factors, the positive factor was the tendency toward biological explanations of mental illness by new researchers, which lessened family guilt and made it possible for family members to come out of the closet about their relative's illness.

NAMI is a product of the present era, one in which the growth of self-help and advocacy groups is truly ubiquitous. The number and variety of self-help groups increase daily, which says something about the kind of society we live in. Whatever social forces explain these other movements must also help explain the growth of NAMI.

Many social scientists agree that self-help movements are signals that society's traditional ways of doing things are not working. The emergence of these new groups provides new ways of solving problems; they focus on peer support and education and rely less heavily on professionals and agencies. There is a recognition that professionals are not omnipotent and that the medical community has limited capacity to provide the range of human support that people need (Back et al. 1976; Caplan and Killilea 1976; Gussow 1976; Tracy and Gussow 1976).

Some writers, for example, Vattano (1972) and Gartner and Riessman (1977), see self-help movements as antibureaucratic, power-to-the-people movements, a true expression of the democratic ideal that acknowledges individuals' capacities to help one another rather than depend excessively on professionals. These movements seem to be a reaction against our culture's traditional reliance on a hierarchy of experts who are supposed to know how to resolve the problems of consumers and against the passivity with which consumers were expected to follow the dictates of the professional. Now there is a challenge to the indiscriminate reliance on professional help, which sometimes produces its own iatrogenic difficulties (Hollander 1980). Gartner (1976) believes that the whole nature and practice of human service provision has come under question. He quoted Margaret Mead as saying there is a "revolt of all people that are being done good to" and that we are at the end of an era in which we thought professionals always knew best.

NAMI appears to be very much in the genre of the self-help movements as they have spread across the country. NAMI now has about 900 local and state affiliates, which includes about 100,000 family members plus interested professionals and other supporters of the organization. To the extent the present rate of growth continues (12–15 new alliances each month) and the organization fully capitalizes on the talents of its members and brings its collective energies to bear on problems at hand, it can be expected to possess considerable clout in the mental health field. It is no longer possible to plan services for the mentally ill nor for programs for families without NAMI's full involvement. The fact that the curriculum and training committee of NAMI can today bring together at a national conference some of the most recognized figures in family treatment testifies to the fact that NAMI has truly arrived on the mental health scene.

CURRENT ISSUES IN COST OF SERVICES

No matter what we propose by way of help to families, we cannot avoid the issue of cost per unit of service. One of the most perplexing issues of our time is how to reduce the cost of care for physical and mental health treatment. There are high-level discussions and much rethinking by government, employees, providers, insurance carriers, and consumers as to how our society can afford to provide all the services that Americans have come to believe they are entitled to. Changes are certainly in the wind, and providers and service users must stay abreast of what is happening.

Frank and Kamlett (1985) have estimated, using figures from the mental health sector, the general medical sector, and the human service sector including transportation costs and transfer of payments, that the direct costs and expenditures for mental health care in 1980 ranged between $19.2 and $22 billion. It is unlikely that that sum will decrease much in the near future; therefore, the utmost in cost consciousness will be required. Choices will have to be made. Money spent to give support and training to families may not be available for the residential care for patients for which many families aspire.

There was a time when medical insurance seemed to cover most health needs, and to a lesser extent mental health needs, that consumers identified, and few among us ever expected that significant change was likely. But things are changing, and it is important to note what some of these changes are and why they are occurring.

Among those highly concerned are employers. Employers found it to their advantage to offer to their employees significant fringe benefits as part of their total actual earnings, which served as a good tax break to employers. Among the most important fringe benefits, of course, was health insurance. Problems arose because costs to insurers began rising so fast, up 24.25% per year in many Blue Cross plans. The reasons for this were the stimulated demands for service and the increased charge per unit of service (Talbott and Dauner 1985). Employers have become concerned because of the greatly increased costs to them. Consumers are upset because they are required to pay higher deductibles and higher premiums. Changes in how insurance is to be provided are going to be most strongly influenced by buyers of care—large employers and their employees. The system has changed, Talbott and Dauner (1985) advise, from one driven by decisions made by physicians, hospitals, Blue Cross/Blue Shield plans, and other large insurers to a system driven by the consuming public. Buyers of care are going to determine how their benefits are structured and how they are going to pay for them. People will need to understand, or course, that there will inevitably be trade-offs between costs and amount of coverage. Consumers are going to be much more cost conscious, and it behooves people offering training to mental health professionals to be aware that what is reimbursable may change drastically. For example, there may be a movement to cover only the truly mentally ill under health insurance. That would mean help to families would not be a reimbursable expense; therefore, help must be kept low in cost, and costs must be met some other way.

Although there are a great number of other issues arising in the area of cost of care, they are beyond our discussion here. The only other fascinating development to be discussed very briefly in this chapter is the trend toward corporate medicine. As Beach (1985) sees it, corporate medicine tends to take one of four directions: 1) several physicians may join to incorporate their practice; 2) other physicians belong to group practices such as health maintenance organizations (HMOs); 3) some hospitals are being acquired by major chains; and 4) some hospitals have split off various functions into private companies. For-profit corporate multihospital ownerships such as Hospital Corporation of America show such good profit margins that much excitement is shown in the financial sections of the *New York Times* and the *Wall Street Journal*. Presumably, corporate medicine has a competitive edge in using personnel economically (Gaylin 1985).

Gaylin (1985) feels that we are truly entering a new era in health care: "It is striking that so many historical trends, some going back as far as 70 years, should mature and converge as dramatically as they have in the last few years. The pressure for change is so strong, it so specific in direction, and has reached such critical levels that it is no longer a question of whether it is bad or good; the trend cannot be halted" (p. 158). Further, he said that "innovative change in psychiatric programming by prepaid groups, for example, could be explosive" (p. 158). The direction is more than formerly toward the HMO and public clinic and much less toward individual private psychotherapy. The HMOs will probably improve services to the mentally ill to improve their competitive edge. The private practitioner, Gaylin informs us, will find himself or herself in a difficult position.

Thus, as we approach the problem of help to families, we are necessarily faced with the question of how services can be paid for. This is difficult because of rapid changes in the way services can be provided, fiscal restraint in government, and the unsettled insurance picture. However uncomfortable these factors make us, we cannot wish them away. Planning help for families must be done within these realities.

SUMMARY AND CONCLUSIONS

For the first time there is a national focus on families who are affected by relatives who have mental illnesses. Many articles have reported on the experiences of families and their aspirations and needs, and from it all, new direction in providing help will emerge. The purpose of this chapter is, to the extent possible, to place the issue of help giving in the context of our times. Several considerations seem crucial and most of them need more study. First, there are American traditions, customs, and laws that set parameters around what is permissible. Then there is the subculture with which families are in close contact—the mental health care system—which has its own ideologies and conventions that are difficult to influence. However, new on the scene are a couple of forces that spell change. There is the emerging consumer advocacy movement, bringing its growing political clout to bear on a system of care that needs considerable change. Finally, there is the reality of costs of service that are no longer willingly borne by insurance carriers or taxpayers, necessitating careful scrutiny of cost/benefit ratios in everything we do.

REFERENCES

Bachrach LL: The chronic patient: sociological thought in psychiatric care. Hosp Community Psychiatry 38:819–820, 1987

Back KW, Taylor RC: Self-help groups: tool or symbol. Journal of Applied Behavioral Science 12:295–309, 1976

Bayer R: Homosexuality and American Psychiatry: The Politics of Diagnosis. New York, Basic Books, 1981

Beach W: Corporate medicine. Hosp Community Psychiatry 36:113, 1985

Caplan G, Killilea M (eds): Support Systems and Mutual Help: Interdisciplinary Explorations. New York, Grune & Stratton, 1976

Chesler P: Women and Madness. Garden City, NY, Doubleday, 1972

Frank R, Kamlett M: Direct costs and expenditures for mental health care in the United States in 1980. Hosp Community Psychiatry 36:165–167, 1985

Gartner A: The Preparation of Human Service Professionals. New York, Human Services Press, 1976

Gartner A, Riessman F: Self-help in the Human Services. San Francisco, CA, Jossey-Bass, 1977

Gaylin S: The coming of the corporation and the marketing of psychiatry. Hosp Community Psychiatry 36:154–159, 1985

Gussow Z: The role of self-help clubs in adaptation to chronic illness and disability. Soc Sci Med 10:407–414, 1976

Harshbarger D: The human service organization, in A Handbook of Human Service Organizations. Edited by Demone HW, Harshbarger D. New York, Human Sciences Press, 1978, pp 22–31

Hatfield AB: Psychological costs of schizophrenia to the family. Social Work 23:355–359, 1978

Hatfield AB: The family as partner in the treatment of mental illness. Hosp Community Psychiatry 30:338–340, 1979

Hatfield AB, Lefley HP (eds): Families of the Mentally Ill: Coping and Adaptation. New York, Guilford, 1987

Hatfield A, Spaniol L, Zipple A: Expressed emotion: a family perspective. Schizophr Bull 13:221–226, 1987

Hersch C: Social history, mental health, and community control. Am Psychol 27:749–753, 1972

Holden DH, Lewine RJ: How families evaluate mental health professionals, resources, and effects of illness. Schizophr Bull 8:626–633, 1982

Hollander R: A new service ideology: the third mental health revolution. Professional Psychology 11:561–566, 1980

Illich I: Medical Nemesis. New York, Pantheon, 1975

Illich I: Disabling Professions. London, Marion Boyers, 1977

Klein J: The least restrictive alternative: more about less. Psychiatr Q 55:106–114, 1983

Lefley HP: Aging parents as caregivers of mentally ill adult children: an emerging social problem. Hosp Community Psychiatry 38:1063–1070, 1987

Levine M: The History and Politics of Community Mental Health. New York, Oxford University Press, 1981

McKnight J: The professional service business. Social Policy 8:110–116, 1977

Morris R: Overcoming cultural and professional myopia in education for the human services, in A Handbook of Human Service Organizations. Edited by Demone HW, Harshbarger D. New York, Human Sciences Press, 1978, pp 233–248

National Alliance for the Mentally Ill: Advocacy for persons with chronic mental illness: building a nationwide network. Proceedings of the 1979 national conference of the National Alliance for the Mentally Ill, Rosslyn, VA, 1979

Penfold PS, Walker GA: Women and the Psychiatric Paradox. Montreal, Eden Press, 1983

Potasznik H, Nelson G: Stress and social support: the burden experienced by the family of a mentally ill person. Am J Community Psychol 12:589–607, 1984

Ritvo E: Primary responsibility: with whom should it rest? in Autism: Diagnosis, Current Research, and Management. Edited by Ritvo E. New York, Spectrum, 1976

Rochefort DA: Origins of the "third psychiatric revolution": the community mental health centers act. J Health Polit Policy Law 9:1–30, 1984

Sarason SB: Psychology Misdirected. New York, Free Press, 1981

Talbott J, Dauner MR: An insurance executive looks at changing patterns of health care: an interview with Marlon R. Dauner. Hosp Community Psychiatry 36:160–164, 1985

Torrey EF: Surviving Schizophrenia: A Family Manual. New York, Harper & Row, 1983

Tracy CS, Gussow Z: Self-help groups: a grass roots response to needs for services. Journal of Applied Behavioral Science 12:310–316, 1976

Vattano AJ: Power to the people: self-help group. Social Work 17:7–15, 1972

The Disabled Family

Leona L. Bachrach, Ph.D.

For numerous years I have been devoting considerable energy to analyzing the problems that are associated with the planning and delivery of adequate, relevant, and humane services for chronic mental patients. Although I am a sociologist by training and am not involved in the provision of direct services to these patients, I am very deeply committed to their care. I have never considered myself to be, nor would I ever want to be, a mere bystander. Accordingly, I have attempted over the years to keep up with new problems in service delivery as they emerge and with new solutions as they are presented.

During the time that services for chronic mental patients have so preoccupied me, I have witnessed the birth and the phenomenal growth of a strong family movement in the United States—an important development in the history of service planning and one that I applaud as a major step in the right direction. Dr. Hatfield's chapter eloquently charts the social significance of that movement, and, for that reason alone, it is an extremely worthwhile discussion.

But that is hardly the entire significance of Dr. Hatfield's contribution. Her chapter also provides an opportunity—one that I cannot resist—to bridge the gap between academically oriented concepts in service planning and the real world of service delivery as it is experienced by families of the chronically mentally ill. In the space that has been allotted to me, I will capitalize on that opportunity. I shall not attempt to either paraphrase the substance of Dr. Hatfield's remarks or take issue with the points that she raises. Indeed, that would be both difficult and foolhardy! Instead, I shall attempt to expand on her excellent sociological analysis of the cultural context within which families of the chronically mentally ill must seek help and guidance as they attempt to deal with the overwhelming needs of their disabled relatives.

SOURCES OF DISABILITIES

The word *disabled* is a key concept in my response to Dr. Hatfield's chapter. I should like to start out by noting, simply, that the noun *disability* also has a verb form—*to disable*. That disability is a process is something that I suspect we tend to forget. To disable, according to Webster (1972), is to render an individual unfit, unable, or incapacitated. If one thinks of disability in this way—as a dynamic process instead of as a static condition that characterizes the chronically ill patient—one may begin to perceive the patient as an individual who has been rendered unfit, unable, or incapacitated by certain circumstances that are associated, either directly or indirectly, with his or her illness.

As I read Dr. Hatfield's chapter, I was struck by the notion that the concept of disability is hardly limited to patients. It is also exquisitely descriptive of what happens to the families of those patients, who, in an analogous manner, are rendered unfit, unable, or incapacitated by the circumstances of their relatives' illnesses. And it is the disability of families, their incapacity to deal with the demands generated by their relatives' illnesses, on which I want to focus my brief remarks.

In fact, this analogy, even though it is obviously metaphorical in a number of ways, is a most productive one. An understanding of the nature of disability—of its sources and dynamics—can provide an excellent context within which to analyze the concerns raised by Dr. Hatfield.

Shepherd (1984) and Wing and Morris (1981) in Great Britain distinguish among three essential varieties of disability affecting the chronically mentally ill: primary, secondary, and tertiary disability. It is my contention that there are certain parallels between patients and their families in the experience of these disabilities; although, as I said, the analogy is incomplete.

Primary Disability

The first level of disability described by these authors is primary disability, and I want to deal with that one quickly because the analogy is weakest here. Primary disability is the most clinically "pure" type. It consists of psychiatric impairments or dysfunctions that may otherwise be described as symptoms of illness. For example, in the case of people with schizophrenia, primary disabilities might include such conditions as lethargy, odd and unacceptable behavior, a lack of awareness of handicaps, and disturbances in social relationships. It is typically the appearance of these primary disabilities that leads to diagnosis and, for many chronically mentally ill people, to engagement with the mental health service system.

There is, of course, no direct parallel for primary disability among families. Because families are not themselves ill, they obviously do not themselves have primary disabilities. But there is a sociological circumstance that we need to consider: Dr. Hatfield points out in numerous places in her presentation that even though the family is not ill, service providers and service systems nonetheless often behave as if primary disability resides in the family. That is, families of the chronically mentally ill continue to be condemned for schizophrenogenesis—and that is a clue to the sociological forces that propel the system of care.

Secondary Disability

But I would like to move on to what the British authors refer to as secondary disabilities, which are more to the point I want to make. I believe that these secondary disabilities have direct parallels for patients and families. Secondary disabilities stem from handicaps that are associated with the *experience* of illness, and not with the illness per se. Wing and Morris (1981) referred to secondary disabilities as "adverse personal reactions," and Shepherd (1984) aptly reminded us that "a major psychiatric episode is a frightening and disturbing experience and its effects may persist long after the primary symptoms have disappeared" (p. 5). Secondary disabilities, in short, represent an individual's idiosyncratic responses to illness.

The range of possible secondary disabilities for chronically mentally ill individuals is very great, simply because the number of idiosyncratic responses to the experience of psychiatric illness is probably almost limitless. However, some typical examples of secondary disabilities among patients might include responses of wariness, avoidance, and withdrawal, as well as refusal to accept the limits of illness and persistent clinging to unrealistic goals. The presence of these secondary disabilities may present as much of a problem for successful engagement and treatment as do the primary symptoms of the illness.

It does not take extraordinary powers of analysis to recognize that these kinds of responses similarly characterize the families of the chronically mentally ill. Dr. Hatfield pointed out much more eloquently than I can that the emergence of serious and apparently irreversible illness in a family member overwhelms and victimizes his or her relatives. There is probably no such thing as being prepared for the appearance of the illness, and it is not surprising that many relatives respond with wariness and withdrawal. Indeed, one of the primary de facto functions of the family movement is helping family members to accept the limits imposed by their relatives' illness and to abandon unrealistic goals on behalf of those individuals.

Tertiary Disability

Tertiary disabilities similarly characterize both chronically mentally ill individuals and their family members. What distinguishes this class of disabilities from the primary and secondary ones is that they have their genesis in societal reactions. Thus, Wing and Morris (1981) referred to tertiary disabilities as "social disablements" that derive from societal responses to illness and incapacity. For patients, tertiary disabilities typically include such circumstances as diminished social networks, poverty, unemployment, and a general lack of belonging. Once established, these tertiary disabilities tend to persist over time and to culminate in a distinct social disadvantage for the chronically mentally ill.

Once again, a similar array of tertiary disabilities may be seen to affect the families of the chronically mentally ill. They too experience diminished social networks as they face the enormous burden of providing care for their ill relatives. They must seek, but often find only with great difficulty (if at all), surrogate social supports. If they were not in poverty before illness struck, they soon find themselves victimized by the economics of having a chronically ill dependent—a situation ably discussed by Dr. Hatfield.

Indeed, I would go so far as to suggest that tertiary disabilities constitute a major portion of what is now called family burden. And, once again, the family movement serves to ease some of that very heavy load as it is experienced by families of the chronically mentally ill.

Societal Pressures and Expectations

Although I believe that the British experts to whom I have been referring do an admirable job of sorting out the origins and complexities of disability among the chronically mentally ill—and, by extension, among their families—I should like to add another dimension to their conceptualizations by noting an additional kind of disability to which both chronic mental patients and their families are typically exposed. I am referring now to social circumstances that are over and above tertiary disabilities; they are more general aspects of social life that may potentially affect any individual, and they are not related to illness per se. Society, in short, frequently provides expectations and standards that in some way incapacitate individuals. And, because the chronically mentally ill and their families are also humans, they too encounter societal pressures and expectations that are limiting and at times even disabling. The major difference, of course, is that for the chronically mentally ill and their families, the ensuing disabilities are so grave, so persistent, and so ubiquitous that they tend to become the central realities of life.

Thus, professional infighting among the different disciplines involved in the treatment of the mentally ill is perhaps, by some standards, par for the course. Why should the delivery of mental health services be subjected to standards that are different from those characterizing other concerns in American life? Why should it matter so much that the pluralism, territoriality, and guild interests, which are so ably described by Dr. Hatfield, predominate? The answer, of course, lies not in any intrinsic fault with professional self-interest, which is amply rewarded in our culture, but rather in the severe burden that this imposes on people who are already severely disabled by the effects of chronic mental illness.

INTERACTION OF SOURCES OF DISABILITY

It is much easier to identify these various sources of disability in the abstract than it is to tie them definitively to real-life circumstances. Perhaps the example of homelessness among the chronically mentally ill will suffice for illustrative purposes. In recent months, considerable attention has been focused on this topic (Bachrach 1984a, 1984b; Lamb 1984), and it is a source of major professional concern.

A review of the current literature on the homeless mentally ill leads unequivocally to the conclusion that homelessness within this population may be related to a wide range of disabilities that are associated with chronic mental illness (Bachrach 1986a). Thus, for some people who are chronically mentally ill, homelessness is clearly an expression of a secondary disability: the wariness and paranoia that characterize many of these individuals probably stem directly from their idiosyncratic responses to their illnesses. However, for other members of the chronically mentally ill population, homelessness may more nearly be a tertiary disability. In fact, Wing and Morris (1981) specifically mention homelessness as one kind of tertiary disability that accompanies poverty, stigma, and other societal responses to the presence of chronically mentally ill people. And certainly such greater societal pressures as urban gentrification contribute materially to homelessness for some mentally ill individuals. In specific cases, however, homelessness probably often results from a complicated interaction of many sources of disability.

The example of homelessness thus serves to underscore two important points: 1) the absence of domicile among the chronically mentally ill has more than one cause, and effective planning must be tuned in to the multiplicity of antecedents; and 2) in the case of any given mentally ill individual, many circumstances—a combination of primary, secondary, and tertiary disabilities as well as external societal pressures—probably interact in a complex manner to create or to support the condition, so that there are no simple solutions.

Similarly, various kinds of disabilities interact in complex ways to create frustration and helplessness among families of chronically mentally ill individuals. Families must stand by and watch their loved ones progress through the stages of their illnesses. They must modify expectations and hopes for their children or spouses. They must deal with real-world tertiary disabilities like inadequate programs, insufficient funds, and low program priorities. They must learn to live with professional infighting and bureaucratic inefficiencies that take on exceptional consequences in the face of their other frustrations and fears. It appears, then, that helplessness—disability—among the families of the chronically mentally ill is fueled by multiple circumstances and is often, seemingly, practically boundless.

THE FAMILY MOVEMENT IN REDUCING SOURCES OF DISABILITY

I have alluded to the family movement as a disability-reduction initiative several times during the course of these remarks. I believe that the family movement does in fact have a critical role to play in reducing, or even eliminating, some of the sources of disability that family members typically endure. In the area of secondary disability, for example, the family movement serves to lend education, support, and realistic hope to the relatives of very sick people at a time when they most need it. In the area of tertiary disability, the family movement often pursues efforts to reduce stigma and also pursues such pragmatic goals as eliminating restrictive covenants. And merely by lending mutual support, the family movement helps families to overcome societally engendered disabilities that exacerbate their vulnerability and defenselessness. Even in the area of primary disability, the family movement lends important disability-reduction services through its unflagging support of basic research.

In fact, I would carry my comments a step further. Not only is the family movement important in the reduction and elimination of disability among families of the chronically mentally ill, today it is absolutely essential. In an era when programs supporting chronic mental patients are being terminated much more rapidly than new programs are being developed (Bachrach 1986b), in an era when the nation's demographic structure is leading to increased numbers of young chronically mentally ill individuals with anticipated long periods of dependency (Bachrach 1982, 1984c), the mutual support and legal advocacy of the family movement are necessary for the very survival of those families.

In the end, of course, this can only hold great benefit for mentally ill people themselves, for, as Dr. Hatfield so ably demonstrated, they are ultimately dependent on their families as their major source of support. Strong patients who are able to combat their many disabilities need strong families who can combat theirs.

REFERENCES

Bachrach LL: Young adult chronic patients: an analytical review of the literature. Hosp Community Psychiatry 33:189–197, 1982

Bachrach LL: Interpreting research on the homeless mentally ill: some caveats. Hosp Community Psychiatry 35:914–917, 1984a

Bachrach LL: Research on services for the homeless mentally ill. Hosp Community Psychiatry 35:910–913, 1984b

Bachrach LL: The young adult chronic psychiatric patient in an era of deinstitutionalization. Am J Public Health 74:382–384, 1984c

Bachrach LL: The context of care for the chronic mental patient with substance abuse problems. Psychiatr Q 58:3–14, 1986a

Bachrach LL: The future of the state mental hospital. Hosp Community Psychiatry 37:467–474, 1986b

Lamb HR (ed): The Homeless Mentally Ill. Washington, DC, American Psychiatric Association, 1984

Shepherd G: Institutional Care and Rehabilitation. London, Longman, 1984

Webster's New World Dictionary of the English Language, 2nd College Edition. New York, World Publishing, 1972, p 400

Wing JK, Morris B: Clinical basis of rehabilitation, in Handbook of Psychiatric Rehabilitation. Edited by Wing JK, Morris B. Oxford, Oxford University Press, 1981, pp 3–16

Chapter 4

Family-Provider Relationships: Charting a New Course

Kayla F. Bernheim, Ph.D.

David is a 20-year-old man who has been recently discharged from the psychiatric ward of his local hospital. When he was admitted, he had been hearing voices and had had some unrealistic ideas about the young woman who lived across the street. Believing that she was being held prisoner, and that she was waiting for him to save her (a message that he believed to have been telepathically sent), he broke into her home and was arrested. David spent 2 months in the hospital, where he received antipsychotic medications and supportive contact with hospital staff. His parents were asked to provide a social history for the records, were told to feel free to visit him regularly but to stay for brief periods of time, and were notified by the social worker that David would be coming home 4 days before his scheduled discharge.

On his return home, David showed his parents his prescription. Although he did not want to have it filled, his parents insisted. For weeks, he stayed to himself almost all the time, coming out of his room only for meals. He seemed to have no interest in anything. He looked like a zombie, and indeed, he complained that the medicine made him feel empty. David's parents tried to call the doctor, but their call was routed instead to the social worker who told them the medicine was necessary to keep David well, that he would probably have to take it for years, and that the doctor would see David every 3 months and make any changes that were necessary. Ten days later, heartsick at the change in their son, and tired of hearing his continuous complaints about the medicine, they agreed that he should stop taking it and see how he did on his own. Six weeks later he relapsed and returned to the hospital.

99

Susan is a 21-year-old sophomore in college. Like David, she had had a psychotic episode from which she had recovered fairly well with hospitalization and medication. Preparatory to discharge, the treatment team suggested that Susan consider living in a halfway house and attending the hospital's day program for several months before returning to school. Her parents were appalled—surely Susan could not benefit from associating with the kinds of people whom they had seen in the hospital. To them she seemed back to her old self, and they were concerned that if she didn't go back to college now, she might become too frightened to go back at all. Besides, she had a whole semester to make up and neither Susan nor her family wanted her to fall behind. Susan, with her family's approval, returned directly to college where she enrolled for a full course load and also made arrangements with her previous professors to make up her "incompletes" by the end of the term. However, she was back in the hospital before the end of the term.

In both scenarios, a failure to prevent relapse occurred. Whereas many, perhaps most, providers would lay these failures at the feet of the families, in our view, they belong to the professionals who neglected to provide the kinds of information and guidance that would have fostered a better outcome. Situations like these occur with maddening frequency—maddening to professionals whose goal is to prevent relapse, maddening to patients who suffer massive assaults to self-esteem with each breakdown, and maddening to family members who wish, above all else, to help their ill relative, be it parent, child, sibling, or spouse, become and remain well. In this chapter, I will explore why such failures to communicate effectively occur and how they can best be prevented.

The ideology of provider-family relationships is still entrenched, to a significant degree, in the era of asylum described by Terkelsen (Chapter 1 of this volume). At that time, due to the fact that patients were not expected to improve, and based on the notion that family life represented some part of the noxious environment from which patients needed protection, families were encouraged to disengage from their ill loved one. Providers and families communicated very little, and indeed, there was scant reason to do so. Today, however, families have come to assume (often by default) a far greater share of the caretaking responsibility for their impaired loved one. They carry this responsibility burdened by the stigma and isolation that accompany mental illness in the family as well as by the inevitable intrafamilial conflicts and emotional drain that the presence of such a person generates. They now need a great deal of support, information, and guidance from professional care givers, many of whom lack the interest and the skills necessary to provide what is needed. As families have been asked to fill a new role, they have asked providers to do so as well. Surveys of families (Hatfield 1978, 1983;

Holden and Lewine 1982) uniformly report that the professional community has been slow to make the needed shift in perspective.

Further, professionals who have taken an interest in working with families of the chronically mentally ill have approached the issue with an incompletely thought-out systems orientation in which the family's impact on the patient is scrutinized but the patient's impact on the family has been neglected almost entirely (Goldstein and Rodnick 1975; Terkelson and Cole 1985). Observing that these families often appear disorganized, conflict ridden, and dysfunctional (when they are interviewed, usually at a time of maximum stress), clinicians with a systems viewpoint have too quickly jumped to the conclusion that the family's dysfunction is contributory (or even causal) to the patient's symptomatology. They have failed to consider an equally obvious conclusion, that the patient's illness (and the social context in which it occurs) is contributory (or even causal) to the family's dysfunction. Family systems assumptions that neglect the wealth of data documenting a biological substrate to the "functional" psychoses have led to a set of interventions, the iatrogenic effects of which are only recently receiving the attention they deserve (Grunebaum 1984; Terkelsen 1983; Hare-Mustin 1980).

The real limitations inherent in the professional community care system and the emerging consumerism of the family movement provide a powerful impetus for providers to reexamine their biases and presuppositions and to struggle toward a more cooperative relationship with families of the chronically mentally ill. If we do not, we will find scenarios like those at the beginning of this chapter repeated endlessly. We will also find that we have alienated our most powerful allies in the struggle to access funds to serve this population of patients whose care has been entrusted to us. The remainder of this chapter will focus on describing the ideal provider-family relationship, discussing how families and providers can be helpful to each other and how both, functioning as a rehabilitation team, can be helpful to patients—as individuals and as a class. We will also take a closer look at some of the barriers to effective collaboration that exist at present.

ASSUMPTIONS

This chapter is predicated on several assumptions that are best made explicit so they can be examined critically. The first assumption is that the great majority of families are motivated to be of service to their impaired members. Much of what is perceived by professionals as disinterest is iatrogenically induced (Bernheim 1982). For example, families whose past contacts with professionals have left them feeling guilty and powerless will quite naturally be reticent to reinvolve themselves. Those who expect to be coerced into accepting a greater share of caretaking responsibility than they would like will, likewise, withdraw protectively. It is further assumed that much of what is perceived as "sabotage" of treatment is the result of ignorance (for example, about medications, negative symptoms, cognitive impairment). Sometimes, in fact, the ignorance lives within the professional who neglects important data that the family has to offer (for example, about prodromal signs, current stresses, and medication side effects). It is assumed that relatives want the patient to be as well as possible, and further, that they are willing to undergo considerable sacrifice to bring this about. This may not seem like a questionable assumption, but, in fact, descriptions of these families in the professional literature have been ubiquitously negative. The assumption of malign (although subconscious, to be sure) intent, while subtly expressed, runs through much of how professionals communicate about these families (see, for example, Haley 1980; Madanes 1981; Lidz 1973). The etiological notions of "psychotic family games" of Selvini-Palazzoli et al. (1989) are a case in point.

The second assumption is that having a chronically impaired (whether physically or emotionally) family member exerts considerable strain on the adaptive capacities of the well members (Hatfield 1978; Lefley 1987). The financial, emotional, and social burden imposed by the illness is currently underassessed but clearly substantial (Goldman 1982). Chronic stress has predictable sequelae that must be ameliorated if the family and patient are to function maximally.

The third assumption is that chronic mental illnesses are, by and large, biological conditions (Henn and Nasrallah 1982; Paykel 1982). This assumption is supported by a great deal of data with respect to the schizophrenias, major affective disorders, and, of course, psychotic disorders with clearly organic bases. These conditions produce, among other symptoms, characteristic cognitive deficits, the amelioration of which requires a specialized environment. For example, the environment that is most supportive of maximum functioning for a recovering schizophrenic person is generally high in structure and clarity, and low in quantity and intensity of stimulation.

It can be seen that the third assumption, combined with the second, places families on the horns of a dilemma. Often, the presence of chronic mental illness in the family, particularly when accompanied by a lack of understanding of the nature of the patient's deficits, increases stress and decreases clarity when just the opposite would be beneficial. Indeed, the surprising aspect of the data on "expressed emotion" (Brown et al. 1972; Vaughn and Leff 1976; Vaughn et al 1984; Goldstein and Doane 1982) is not that some families are unable to provide a rehabilitative environment, but rather that so many families have been able to do so, on their own, with little guidance or support from indigenous support systems or from mental health professionals.

This leads to the fourth assumption, which is that developing such a specialized environment requires specialized knowledge and skills that families do not ordinarily possess. Families of the chronically mentally ill are much like other families—some are noisy, busy, and emotionally expressive, others are quiet, sedate, and emotionally restrained, and most have styles somewhere in between. There is nothing abnormal about any of these styles; however, some suit the special needs of chronically mentally ill patients better than others. These styles may well be modifiable, within limits, but only when families have a conceptual framework within which change can be understood. Many families have developed this understanding themselves, pragmatically, in piecemeal fashion, through trial and error. Many more could be helped to do so.

The fifth assumption is that family members must often make decisions about treatment strategies for their ill family member and for themselves. Although the issue of who should make choices for a person whose judgment is impaired is far from resolved, families are often in a position of influence even when they are not in a position of direct power, as in the two case examples offered at the beginning of this chapter. Further, the principle of informed consent is embedded within the system of medical ethics but is often neglected when it comes to family work (Hare-Mustin et al. 1979; McElroy, Chapter 6 of this volume). It cannot be assumed that family therapy has no negative outcomes (Graziano and Fink 1973; Hare-Mustin 1980; Terkelsen 1983). Families need a great deal of information about their relative's illness and their own rights and responsibilities to make truly informed choices, and it is the professional's obligation to provide this information.

The final assumption is that the professional mental health community has failed to meet the needs of families in a way that would allow them to maximally fulfill their responsibilities to themselves and to their impaired member. By and large, providers lack both the conceptual framework and the skills necessary to educate and collaborate effectively with families. For the next generation of mental health practitioners to do a better job than the current one has done, substantial changes in curriculum and training are required.

FEATURES OF A COOPERATIVE ALLIANCE

Open and ongoing communication is, of course, essential to cooperation between any participants with respect to any task. Too often family members are seen to acquire a social history and are not contacted again (if at all) until their relative is about to be discharged from the institution or agency. Further, families report not having telephone calls returned, being shunted from one member of the treatment team to another, being made to feel that their questions and concerns are inappropriate intrusions into the therapeutic arena, and, in general, being ignored by providers.

Even well-intentioned professionals are liable to leave the task of initiating contact up to the family, particularly when other issues seem to require more immediate attention. We cannot assume that if families do not call us, they do not want or need our help, or that they are unwilling to participate in rehabilitation activities. They may harbor a host of expectations (some of which may have been iatrogenically induced) that prevent their doing so despite dire need or benevolent motives.

Creating channels of communication could take a multitude of forms including, but certainly not restricted to, setting aside regular office hours for telephone contact with families, specifying a family ombudsman from among the members of the treatment team, or holding informational workshops. Doing so, however, requires a profound change in attitude: we must learn to acknowledge both the family's rights as consumers and capacities as partners in rehabilitation.

The ideal family-provider relationship is also characterized by mutual respect and a reasonably equal balance of power. As we ask families to acknowledge our expertise, we should also acknowledge theirs. As we teach, so should we learn. As we ask families to accept our role as decision makers, we should accept that they too have this role.

Decisions that affect the patient who lives at home also affect the family. For example, who will provide transportation to a day program? How does the patient's social withdrawal affect the ambiance of the household? How will the parents negotiate disagreements about how the patient's symptoms should be managed? How will the family manage financially if the patient is responsible for his or her own funds and spends his or her social security disability check on cigarettes and video games? In this situation, close collaboration between the provider and family seems ethically mandatory.

Professionals also need to learn that families can disagree with professional recommendations—they do not always "deny," "resist," or "sabotage." Disrespectful language reflects disrespectful attitudes (Lewine 1983).

Families of the chronically mentally ill can collaborate with providers on systemic as well as individual issues. Whereas professionals can hardly advocate for money for programs and services without appearing self-serving, families can represent the needs of this often-overlooked group of citizens with far greater effectiveness. Precedent for this role has been set by families of retarded citizens whose concerted lobbying has brought about a revolution in the care of their loved ones.

Families can also serve a watchdog function. For example, at Northampton State Hospital in Massachusetts a model program uses family monitors to provide information about ward activities, safety, and treatment to administrative staff (Reiter and Plotkin 1985). Over time, ward staff learned to view these family members as allies rather than as adversaries. Families' groups may also be instrumental in evaluating the cost-effectiveness of various treatment options, advocating for those that have proven value and against those that are wasteful or ineffective. In this capacity, they can provide the impetus for creative use of the limited dollars available to serve this population.

WHAT PROFESSIONALS CAN OFFER FAMILIES

What families want from providers is well documented (Hatfield 1983; Holden and Lewine 1982) and dovetails nicely with recent data suggesting that relapse can be prevented through family intervention (Kopeikin 1981; Falloon et al. 1984; Hogarty et al. 1986). First, and most important, providers can educate families about the symptoms, causes, treatments, and prognosis of the patient's illness. This essentially didactic function accomplishes several goals. First, by acknowledging that the patient's illness reflects a biochemical defect, the family is absolved (at least to some extent) of debilitating guilt and obsessive ruminating about fantasized catastrophic errors in parenting. Family members are also less likely to overindulge the patient in an attempt to "pay back" for past mistakes and are generally less frustrated and angry with him or her when they are able to distinguish between behaviors that are symptoms and those that are under voluntary control. As they gain an understanding of the cognitive and emotional deficits their loved one experiences, they are able to set more realistic expectations, based on current level of functioning rather than on the hopes and dreams they had before the onset of illness. Further, they are able to refine their monitoring skills so that their natural vigilance can be put to maximum use if the patient becomes ill again. In this context, they need to be taught (or helped to deduce from their own experience) what signs and symptoms are predictive of relapse for their relative.

Families find it helpful to be given a conceptual framework that can guide their behavior (Bernheim and Lehman 1985a). For example, the stimulus-overload model of schizophrenia, which is consistent with phenomenological accounts by patients (MacDonald 1960) and also with what is known about the brain biochemistry of this illness (Andreasen 1984), helps family members to understand why a quiet, structured environment characterized by simplicity, predictability, and clarity is optimal for patients with this diagnosis. It also helps them to understand that the so-called negative symptoms may serve a protective function for patients who are easily overwhelmed. They learn to be more tolerant of their relative's need for interpersonal distance. Operating within this framework, they are better able to generalize suggestions that are offered, as well as to generate their own solutions to the problem of environmental stress.

The model also provides a rationale for medication. Families need to understand why medication is being prescribed, how it works, that it generally suppresses symptoms rather than curing the illness, and what side effects it generally causes. Once they understand that finding the right medication at the right dosage is a trial-and-error process that can take some time, they are often more supportive and realistic. Indeed, they can participate in this process in a meaningful way, as discussed below.

In addition to providing information about the salient features of the illness and its treatment, professionals ought to provide some training and guidance about coping with residual symptoms and the problems of daily living that can be expected to arise. This may involve, in addition to discussing specific situations, offering skills training in a number of areas.

Family members can be helped to develop a style of communicating that is consistent with the cognitive deficits their relative experiences. For example, they can be taught to give simple rather than complex messages, to modulate the intensity and speed of communications, and to avoid emotionally laden exchanges whenever possible. Further, they can share these skills with others with whom the patient interacts and can also organize the noninterpersonal environment so as to maximize predictability and minimize overstimulation.

Because families of the chronically mentally ill are functioning under enormous stress, they may need additional help in developing or shoring up problem-solving skills. The professional can help families anticipate and develop a plan for handling specific situations that are likely to arise (Goldstein and Kopeikin 1981; Kopeikin et al. 1983). These may include coping with violence or suicidal behavior, anticipating upcoming stresses, handling decompensation and rehospitalization, and arranging for their relative's care when they become aged or incapacitated, among many others. Generic training in problem-solving skills can also be valuable as a tool to be used when unanticipated problems arise (Snyder and Liberman 1981).

Behavior management skills can be as useful to families as they are to hospital staff, particularly when the patient lives at home. These strategies can help distinguish between behaviors that are under voluntary control and those that are not. They can bring marginal behaviors under better control. They also afford the family an organized approach to troublesome behaviors, thereby decreasing interpersonal conflict at home and, in addition, providing the patient with a more predictable environment. Providing consistent behavioral outcomes, emphasizing rewards rather than punishments, and learning to shape behavior are skills that must be taught; they are not part of most families' natural repertoire.

Stress management skills can also be taught to family members with good effects. Learning (or relearning) to use exercise, hobbies, socializing, relaxation exercises, cognitive imagery, meditation, and related techniques often helps to minimize the deleterious effects of chronic mental illness within the family.

Not all families will need or want all of the interventions described above. Ideally, we would envision an initial assessment of every patient's family to find out what their strengths and interests are and to develop an individualized plan for helping them achieve whatever their own goals are with respect to their loved one's illness and rehabilitation. Although each agency might be unable to offer each service, an array of services might be made available regionally, including short-term educational groups, skills-training options, and longer-term supportive services. In any case, each family's plan should evolve from an understanding of the needs of the members rather than being applied programmatically as if all families were the same.

The phenomenon of professional "burnout" is well recognized, but has rarely been applied to indigenous caretakers. Powerlessness, helplessness, and fatigue are common features of these families, as they are among families of the chronically medically ill (Brody 1985; Pinkston and Linsk 1984; Cantor 1983). Therefore, providers can be most helpful in fostering a self-help support network by bringing together families with whom they work with other families in similar situations. This is, in fact, one of the primary goals families have for their contact with professionals (Hatfield 1983). The National Alliance for the Mentally Ill and its hundreds of local affiliates are enormously supportive to member families with respect to emotional and practical issues. Providers can refer families to nearby affiliates (or better yet, accompany them to a meeting), help to establish new groups where none exist close by, and teach newly forming groups some leadership, advocacy, and group development skills. It is important for professionals to avoid usurping the leadership role in such groups so as not to foster dependency or instill "patienthood." Rather, the professional's relationship to the group should be advisory and probably time limited.

Perhaps most important, professionals can offer families a truly collaborative role in rehabilitation efforts. Except in the uncommon situation of a patient who refuses (and who is competent to refuse) to allow family contact with the provider, families should be informed of treatment decisions, their advice should be sought when various strategies are contemplated, and their own needs should be respected when they themselves are affected by decisions. We ought to remember that the privilege of confidentiality resides with the patient, not with the professional. If we act in a way that causes or exacerbates rifts between the patient and the family, we risk alienating a source of potential support for the patient far greater than that the mental health system can provide.

WHAT FAMILIES CAN OFFER PROFESSIONALS

Over and above providing a social history, which is a function with generally recognized value, the family can offer a great deal of information and support to professional providers. They often know what specific signs and symptoms are indicative of impending relapse for their own relative. Although certain general features occur commonly (e.g., changes in sleep patterns, social withdrawal, or agitation), some indicators are idiosyncratic. Going on a diet, refusing to wear eyeglasses, and drinking large quantities of milk are examples of accurate signs that families have pointed out to us. Assuming that early intervention can have a positive impact on the severity and duration of relapse, professionals would do well to learn from the family's experiences and to rely on their ongoing monitoring efforts. Further, mental health professionals tend, quite naturally, to focus on pathology. The family may be able to educate us about what strengths, competencies, and interests their relative has that may be relevant to rehabilitation efforts.

Families can often offer good information about what situations their ill relative handles well or poorly, what environmental circumstances are likely to be perceived by the patient as stressful, and what sorts of management strategies are likely to work in their own situation. We are not suggesting that families are all knowing; indeed, their lack of objectivity will sometimes cloud their judgment. However, my own experience dictates that the family's observations and intuitions should be overridden only with great caution.

Monitoring the patient's response to medication (and other therapeutic efforts) offers another meaningful role for families. Often, they have had years of experience with various medications at various dosages and have an excellent sense of what works best. Therefore, clinicians who are beginning treatment with a chronic patient would do well to pay careful attention to family input. In addition, it makes sense to have the family of each newly diagnosed patient keep a proactive record of medication effects and side effects so that the information can be made available to future providers.

Family members are in an ideal position to function as ancillary therapists if they have the energy, investment, and skills necessary to do so. Whether or not the patient lives at home, the family can serve as the hub of the patient's social support network. In this regard, family members can encourage socialization both within and outside of the family, to the extent that the patient can handle it. They can mobilize friends, peers, church, and others to become and remain involved in a supportive, nonthreatening way. To do this, they will find themselves in the position of educating extended family and community members about the facts of mental illness as they confront head-on the myths and stigma that cloak these illnesses.

Family members can also bolster the patient's self-esteem by arranging success experiences and by attending to signs of progress. They may teach the patient how to avoid or manage stressful situations, break complex tasks into component parts, recognize emerging symptoms, and cope with residual symptoms. They may model and teach social and vocational skills. They may provide incentives for activity, productivity, and achievement.

Families can also support treatment compliance through educating and encouraging the patient with regard to the need for medication and attendance at rehabilitative programs. They may assist the patient in finding, evaluating, and getting to such programs as well. To a great extent, the patient's expectations will reflect those of the family. If they expect too much too soon, the patient may relapse in attempting to meet their goals; if they expect too little, they may unwittingly foster withdrawal and hopelessness. Thus, they play a major role in helping the patient to set realistic goals.

The family may decide to take on an even greater caretaking role by having the patient live at home. This is a difficult decision, and often one that is made for the family with little input from them (see Hatfield, Chapter 3 of this volume, and Lefley 1987). If they do choose this role, they are often able to provide a wealth of data about the patient's ongoing level of functioning, symptomatology, and response to treatment. Further, they are in an ideal position to create (and to teach the patient to create) barriers to overstimulation that can enhance the patient's functioning. They can ameliorate, somewhat, the guilt and shame associated with mental illness by providing a nurturant, accepting environment.

To neglect (or interfere with) the family's willingness and capacity to play a role in fostering the patient's rehabilitation is tantamount to providing inadequate care. Again, I am not implying that all family members will want or will be able to accept these responsibilities, nor am I suggesting that they should. Rather, I mean to point out that the possibility of drawing on the strengths and talents of family members is routinely overlooked in general clinical practice.

BARRIERS TO EFFECTIVE COLLABORATION

Outmoded professional ideologies that view the family as either the enemy to be avoided or the "unidentified patient" to be cured constitute the most formidable barriers to a working partnership with families. Changes in graduate curricula that foster greater sensitivity to the plight, burden, and tasks of families are urgently needed (Bernheim and Lehman 1985b). These can include readings as well as observation and supervised practice in interviewing, counseling, educating, and collaborating with families.

A more insidious ideology is embedded within the medical model. Providers are used to being in a position of power with respect to consumers. Families and patients who request information that is within the professional's province, who question the basis for decisions, who assert their own values, and who demand respect for their own competence are rarely afforded a welcome reception; neither are those who are angry, frustrated, and distrustful (a common presentation among families who have had previous negative experiences with providers). Perhaps this is not surprising when we consider that medical and mental health practitioners are called on daily to make decisions of potentially enormous impact on the basis of a clearly inadequate body of knowledge. The defenses that permit continued functioning in such a situation may be somewhat rigid of necessity. Nonetheless, genuine partnership with families and patients cannot be achieved without the willingness to both give and receive knowledge, and the ability to acknowledge both ignorance and impotence from time to time. Again, peer support and sensitivity to these issues early in professional training are key.

The ideology of chronicity also mitigates against effective collaboration among providers and the chronically mentally ill and their families (Minkoff and Stern 1985). Although recent data suggest that the long-term prognosis is much more hopeful than had been generally thought (Harding et al. 1987), treatment of these patients is not stylish and has generally received low priority in community mental health centers (Kirk and Thenlen 1975; Lamb and Edelson 1976). Further, supportive and educational work with these patients and their families has taken a backseat to more dramatic and interesting dynamic, systemic, or strategic orientations. Emerging data on the effectiveness of psychosocial and psychoeducational techniques will, presumably, modify this ideology in time.

Legal barriers to effective collaboration also exist, specifically laws and codes that govern the confidentiality of patient communications. Although it is hard to imagine that regulations would prevent the family of an acutely psychotic young adult from being informed of his or her hospitalization, diagnosis, and plan for treatment, they have certainly been interpreted in this way. We must attend to formulating these guidelines in a way that works for, rather than against, the patient's best interests even as we attend to protecting his or her civil liberties.

Finally, we must modify the training of young mental health providers to include the kinds of didactic skills that would enable them to effectively educate families. Basic counseling skills should be augmented by skills at delivering educational presentations, assessing what has been learned, use of audiovisual aids, role-playing, and other behavioral and experiential techniques.

REFERENCES

Andreasen N: The Broken Brain. New York, Harper & Row, 1984

Bernheim KF: Supportive family counseling. Schizophr Bull 8:634–641, 1982

Bernheim KF, Lehman AF: Working With Families of the Mentally Ill. New York, WW Norton, 1985a

Bernheim KF, Lehman AF: Teaching mental health trainees to work with families of the chronic mentally ill. Hosp Community Psychiatry 36: 1109–1111, 1985b

Brody EM: Parent care as a normative family stress. Gerontologist 25:19–29, 1985

Brown GW, Birley JLT, Wing JK: Influence of family life on the course of schizophrenic disorder: a replication. Br J Psychiatry 121:241–258, 1972

Cantor MJ: Strain among caregivers: a study of experience in the United States. Gerontologist 23:597–604, 1983

Falloon IRH, Boyd JL, McGill CW, et al: Family Care of Schizophrenia. New York, Guilford, 1984

Goldman HH: Mental illness and family burden. Hosp Community Psychiatry 33:557–559, 1982

Goldstein MJ, Doane JA: Family factors in the onset, course, and treatment of schizophrenic spectrum disorders. J Nerv Ment Dis 170:692–700, 1982

Goldstein MJ, Kopeikin HS: Short- and long-term effects of combining drug and family therapy, in New Developments in Interventions With Families of Schizophrenics (New Directions for Mental Health Services, No 12). Edited by Goldstein MJ. San Francisco, CA, Jossey-Bass, 1981, pp 5–26

Goldstein MJ, Rodnick EH: The family's contribution to the etiology of schizophrenia: current status. Schizophr Bull 14:48–63, 1975

Graziano AM, Fink FS: Second-order effects in mental health treatment. J Consult Psychol 40:356–364, 1973

Grunebaum H: Comments on Terkelsen's "Schizophrenia and the Family: II. Adverse Effects of Family Therapy." Fam Proc 23:421–428, 1984

Haley J: Leaving Home: The Therapy of Disturbed Young People. New York, McGraw-Hill, 1980

Harding C, Zubin J, Strauss J: Chronicity in schizophrenia: fact, partial fact, or artifact. Hosp Community Psychiatry 38:477–486, 1987

Hare-Mustin RT: Family therapy may be dangerous to your health. Professional Psychology 11:935–938, 1980

Hare-Mustin RT, Marecek J, Kaplan AG, et al: Rights of clients, responsibilities of therapists. Am Psychol 34:3–16, 1979

Hatfield AB: Psychological costs of schizophrenia to the family. Social Work 23:355–359, 1978

Hatfield AB: What families want of family therapists, in Family Therapy in Schizophrenia. Edited by McFarlane WR. New York, Guilford, 1983, pp 41–64

Henn FA, Nasrallah HA: Schizophrenia as a Brain Disease. New York, Oxford University Press, 1982

Hogarty G, Anderson CM, Reiss DJ, et al: Family psychoeducation, social skills training, and maintenance chemotherapy in the aftercare treatment of schizophrenia. Arch Gen Psychiatry 43:633–642, 1986

Holden DF, Lewine RRJ: How families evaluate mental health professionals, resources, and effects of illness. Schizophr Bull 8:628–633, 1982

Kirk SA, Thenlen MF: Community mental health myths and the fate of former hospitalized patients. Psychiatry 38:209–217, 1975

Kopeikin HS, Marshall V, Goldstein MJ: Stages and impact of crisis-oriented family therapy in the aftercare of acute schizophrenia, in Family Therapy in Schizophrenia. Edited by McFarlane WR. New York, Guilford, 1983, pp 69–98

Lamb H, Edelson MB: The carrot and the stick: inducing local programs to serve long-term patients. Community Ment Health J 12:137–144, 1976

Lefley HP: Aging parents as caregivers of mentally ill adult children: an emerging social problem. Hosp Community Psychiatry 38:1063–1070, 1987

Lewine RRJ: Parents: mental health professionals' scapegoats, in Changing Families. Edited by Sigel E, Laosa LM. New York, Plenum, 1983, pp 925–933

Lidz T: The Origin and Treatment of Schizophrenic Disorders. New York, Basic Books, 1973

MacDonald N: Living with schizophrenia. Can Med Assoc J 82:218–221, 678–681, 1960

Madanes C: Strategic Family Therapy. San Francisco, CA, Jossey-Bass, 1981

Minkoff K, Stern R: Paradoxes faced by residents being trained in the psychosocial treatment of people with chronic schizophrenia. Hosp Community Psychiatry 36:859–864, 1985

Paykel ES (ed): Handbook of Affective Disorders. New York, Guilford, 1982

Pinkston EM, Linsk NL: Behavioral family intervention with the impaired elderly. Gerontologist 24:576–583, 1984

Reiter MS, Plotkin A: Family members as monitors in a state mental hospital. Hosp Community Psychiatry 36:393–395, 1985

Selvini-Palazzoli MT, Cirillo S, Selvini M, et al: Family Games: General Modes of Psychotic Processes in the Family. New York, WW Norton, 1989

Snyder KS, Liberman RP: Family assessment and intervention with schizophrenics at risk for relapse, in New Developments in Interventions With Families of Schizophrenics (New Directions for Mental Health Services, No 12). Edited by Goldstein MJ. San Francisco, CA, Jossey-Bass, 1981, pp 49–60

Terkelsen KG: Schizophrenia and the family, II: adverse effects of family therapy. Fam Proc 22:191–200, 1983

Terkelsen KG, Cole SA: Methodological flaws in the schizophrenic hypothesis and their implications for mental health services in an era of community care. Unpublished paper, Family Institute of Westchester, Mount Vernon, NY, 1985

Vaughn CE, Leff JP: The influence of family and social factors on the course of psychiatric illness: a comparison of schizophrenic and depressed neurotic patients. Br J Psychiatry 37:409–412, 1976

Vaughn CE, Snyder KS, Jones S, et al: Family factors in schizophrenic relapse. Arch Gen Psychiatry 41:1169–1177, 1984

Care of the Chronically Mentally Ill: Is It Honorable Work?

Carol M. Anderson, Ph.D.

There is good reason to criticize the attitudes and practices of mental health professionals in their treatment of the chronically mentally ill. The stories of David and Susan in Dr. Bernheim's discussion highlight the legitimate and growing concerns of family members and professionals interested in the welfare of mentally ill individuals. Not only are clinical resources inadequately allocated to this population, but training resources are not designed to sensitize professionals to existing problems and needs. Furthermore, there are few good teachers who are reasonable role models for young professionals who wish to learn to work with this population. It is crucial that mental health professionals learn to work collaboratively with patients and families, and that they become able to offer a variety of programs and treatments geared toward the needs and interests of those being served. Clearly, to accomplish these goals, major changes must be made in current training programs. Somehow, training opportunities must be designed that will 1) stimulate a commitment to working with this population, 2) change basic attitudes and assumptions about these patients and the care they require, and 3) provide the skills necessary to relate to and help patients and the significant others who care about them.

Dr. Bernheim outlined some of the necessary content and qualities that should be included in training of this sort. Because these characteristics are so similar to what we believe in and, in fact, have outlined in our proposal for a model training program for psycho-educational work (Anderson et al. 1986), I will concentrate here on why there seems to be a problem with professionals committing themselves to this population and adopting these practical, logical, and potentially helpful interventions.

Although any training program must address both attitudes and skills, it is my belief that the skills needed to work more effectively with families of the chronically ill are easy to teach and easy to adopt. Dealing with attitudes and belief systems is another story. Prevailing attitudes must be challenged and changed or most professionals will not seek or use the skills we see as essential. Once the right attitudes have been inculcated, the necessary skills follow naturally. Three basic attitudinal changes are central to professional acceptance of the new methods of treatment, family-provider relationships, and the resultant training to which we must become committed: 1) placing importance and value on working with the chronically mentally ill, even when a "cure" is not on the horizon; 2) assuming that a view of the person in context is relevant and important in understanding and treating mental illness, without blaming families for the patients' problems; and 3) accepting the notion that the provision of information is a legitimate and powerful way of helping patients and families to cope with mental disorders.

DEALING WITH CHRONICITY

Most professionals want to work with patients who not only get better, but who appreciate and respect their efforts to help. They go into the "therapy business" wanting to fix things, to provide ultimate cures. Nowhere are these hopes and dreams more challenged than in work with the chronically ill. Nothing is easily fixed, and a very high percentage of patients do not welcome professional help. Little is done to prepare trainees for these cold facts. They may read about schizophrenia or manic-depressive disease, but most still begin their clinical work thinking that if they care enough or come up with the right drug or interpretation, or by sheer force of will, they can make patients better. When patients do not get better, or when they get better only to have another episode, these unprepared professionals get angry at patients, hopeless about their own ability to help, or both. Because they begin with inappropriate expectations, they are highly vulnerable to professional burnout. Too many quickly escape to private practice and the treatment of the "worried well," claiming it is not a good use of their time to try to help patients who do not want to be helped or who cannot be treated effectively. They simply choose not to work with chronic patients. This is in part because it is difficult work, but also in part because the implicit values of rapid response and cure have not been challenged.

Adequate training for work with the chronically ill must include helping professionals to come to grips with the limits of their professional influence. This process presents different problems to different professionals. Physicians who are trained to assume authority and to act, if not be, omnipotent, too often have difficulty openly sharing what they know and do not know, forming a relationship based on collaboration and equality, and accepting the limitations of their power and effectiveness. Although social workers and nurses more traditionally have assumed roles of caretaking, not cure, they traditionally also have encouraged unnecessary dependency and have failed to assert themselves in the best interests of patients and families. Furthermore, all disciplines have moved increasingly toward a focus on rapid cures and brief interventions. Few professionals, regardless of discipline, have been trained to expect and handle resistance to treatment and change, relapse or recurrence, and the value of constancy over time. The impact of this inadequate training is exacerbated by the fact that mental health systems and third-party reimbursement policies have implicitly and explicitly placed a value on brief treatment, whether or not it is appropriate to the illness. The implicit message is that if a rapid response is not possible, treatment has failed and should be abandoned. Virtually nothing in the training or experience of any professional supports the development of the vital notion of providing ongoing quality care without encouraging dependency.

Those new to the field of mental health must be exposed to training that will convince them that work with the chronically mentally ill is a legitimate use of their energy and resources. They must be helped to understand that even if we do not have cures or ultimate answers, it is possible to offer to improve the quality of life of these patients and those who care about them; it is possible to alter the course of the illness and to alter the level of distress of those who must live with it. Although no treatment program is going to change the nature of chronic illnesses, dedicating one's life to this work can constitute an honorable and rewarding professional career. We must work to ensure that work with chronic illness will be seen as a valuable ongoing commitment, at least as important as all other specialty areas of psychiatry and mental health. Without this major change in the attitudes and value systems of those who will eventually constitute the health-care team, even the current enthusiasm for providing relatives and patients with education and coping techniques will be short-lived.

RELEVANCE OF THE PERSON IN CONTEXT

It has not been so long since psychiatry was dominated by psychoanalytic views of pathology and its treatment. The psychoanalytically oriented professional tended to view the patient's early life experience and family relationships as primary in the development of illness. According to this view, families of patients with illnesses such as schizophrenia were a destructive influence, and a "parentectomy" was often the treatment of choice. Parents and other family members were excluded from treatment and were not given information about the illness or the treatment. When patients were hospitalized, even visiting was discouraged. In summary, families were blamed, accused, or simply ignored. Early family therapists did little to help. Although they were concerned about families, they also assumed a family-etiology stance and continued to blame families using a new language.

The increased acceptance of schizophrenia and manic-depressive disease as primarily biological disorders seemed to bring with it the promise of a new era of more respectful treatment for family members. In some ways, this has begun to happen. There is, in some circles, less blaming of the family for causing the patient's illness. Unfortunately, several other problems have arisen. Many new biologically oriented professionals have developed tunnel vision in which they see nothing as relevant except the patient's response to medication. They are not interested in the patient's psychosocial or vocational difficulties, and, if the patient is unresponsive to drugs, they consider their obligation or ability to help to be terminated. These professionals are no more interested in the needs, concerns, or problems of family members than their psychoanalytic predecessors. Families remain irrelevant except as they are useful in obtaining historical information and, perhaps, insofar as they can help to ensure medication compliance. Again, professionals fail to see family needs and concerns as relevant and fail to respect the strengths family members must draw on to provide for the primary care of patients over time.

The fact that some of these professionals refer patients to other professionals when drugs are not enough is insufficient to ensure reasonable care. Anyone familiar with medical settings knows that if the doctor does not value a treatment, it either does not get done or decreases in quality as other professionals become contaminated by the physician's attitude. As long as the referral for family work or family education is made with the attitudes, "Get this family off my back," or "Nothing can be done, so you handle it," a situation exists that does not operate in the best interests of comprehensive and quality care for patients.

Nonmedical professionals begin by operating at a serious disadvantage in terms of status, power, and respect in psychiatric systems. In addition, they bring another set of difficulties caused by the assumptions and attitudes developed in their own training. Social workers and family therapists, although somewhat more likely to understand that the family and the rest of the patient's social world is important, also fail to see the total picture. They too often continue to regard the family as relevant in the cause or perpetuation of mental disorders. Although they may at least offer families treatment, their unexamined basic assumptions about etiology cause them to continue to blame families. Furthermore, they remain largely unaware of the contributions of biological factors and are not up-to-date on recent research.

In short, few professionals of any discipline are trained to operate using a total systems perspective. The resultant polarity in the treatment of patients can be at best inconsistent and at worst destructive. We must develop training programs that are based on a systemic perspective that includes respect for biological, psychological, familial, and vocational forces. This does not mean that each professional must be prepared to deliver all treatments. Nonmedical health professionals must learn about biological psychiatry, yet they need not learn to prescribe drugs. Psychiatrists must learn about families, vocational training, and other psychosocial variables, yet they need not actually intervene in every system. Being informed of the relevant issues, however, is essential to genuine respect, interdisciplinary cooperation, and, ultimately, cooperation with families.

INFORMATION AS A POWERFUL INTERVENTION

Perhaps one of the most encouraging advances in the past 10 years has been the increased acceptance of the legitimacy of providing patients and relatives with information about mental illness and how to cope with it more effectively. In many quarters, the provision of educational programs is now regarded as a normal and useful component of mental health services—useful to families and patients in decreasing anxiety, providing direction, and demystifying treatments.

It is important to emphasize, however, that this way of operating is still neither included or valued in most mental health systems. In many training and treatment programs, the view remains that education is superficial, and it should be done, if at all, by a lower-status, peripheral professional with little formal training, supervision, or support, primarily to keep family members from confronting physicians and "wasting" their time.

Even when information is provided to families, it is too often provided with little awareness of the basic educational principles we consider in other educational programs—that is, that people learn best when their anxiety is within manageable limits, that material may have to be repeated more than once, and that participants should be encouraged to share, question, and challenge presenters if knowledge is to be truly integrated and assimilated. In fact, because we know so little, the *process* of the dialogue may be as important as the information exchanged. It goes a long way to establishing more respectful family-provider relationships based on equality and mutual respect. Thus, while we must support these training programs that teach professionals to provide education and information for families, we should be attending to the process as well as the content of those efforts. Unless educational programs are carefully developed and implemented, they will be conducted ineffectually, evaluated inappropriately, found to be ineffective prematurely, and discontinued summarily, as just another therapeutic fad.

RECOMMENDATIONS TO ACCOMPLISH ATTITUDINAL CHANGE

How do we encourage a commitment to and value for working with chronic patients, a respect for the relevance of families and other psychosocial factors, and a value system that places an emphasis on the relevance of information for patients and families provided in an effective and respectful way? I have four basic recommendations.

Provide direct and early exposure to families. I believe major attitudinal changes can be facilitated in all professionals if they are provided with a direct and early exposure to the families of chronically ill patients before they have assumed responsibility for patient care. Professionals in training should have a chance to hear about 1) the pain of having a loved one begin to behave in inexplicable ways; 2) the struggles of trying to manage irrational, bizarre, unpredictable, and even violent behaviors with little or no support; and 3) the frustration of attempting to cope with insensitive or unresponsive professionals and mental health policies. Most importantly, they should hear about these issues before they have become invested in a way of operating with patients and families and before they have already made mistakes that will make them defensive. This early exposure to families would be most effective if it could be provided with built-in "distance" before the neophyte professional is on the spot, having to respond to or handle the problems involved. In this way, it will be more likely that they will be able to hear the problems and concerns of families, be critical of traditional practices, and resist the influence of gurus and writings that present unidimensional and unhelpful views of patients and families.

To accomplish this end, I strongly encourage the use of videotapes and speakers from self-help groups and observation of the interviews of other professionals before assigning new clinicians actual responsibility for patients. New professionals of all disciplines experience too much pressure to provide answers and advice when they hear about painful problems. The fact that they do not have ways to help at this phase of their development, and the fact that there are no answers for some of the problems associated with chronic illness, would lead to excessive frustration and tendencies to "flee the field," if clinical responsibility were to be assigned simultaneously with first exposure to the issues.

Provide a solid understanding of chronic mental illness. Too often training in psychopathology is inadequate or limited to a focus on diagnosis, course, and outcome. Insufficient attention is paid to the deficits that occur as a result of major psychiatric disorders and to what these deficits mean in terms of the ability to function over time. Insufficient attention also is paid to an assessment of patients' and families' assets and strengths that may be exploited in the interest of coping or rehabilitation. Trainees also often are not exposed to a thorough, timely review of the literature. The lack of training attention to providing budding clinicians with a solid understanding of chronic mental illnesses leaves clinicians unprepared to 1) establish reasonable goals and expectations, 2) share with patients and families what is known and not known, and 3) relate with ease and comfort to the questions brought to them by patients, relatives, and colleagues.

Reasonable goals are crucial in avoiding unrealistic promises to patients and families. Goals that are too ambitious can only lead to increased disappointment and frustration. Reasonable goals also are crucial in establishing realistic practices that will not cause professional or relative burnout over time. Thorough and ongoing reviews of the relevant literature not only help professionals to provide adequate information to families, but help to increase their comfort in working collaboratively with families. Genuine competence decreases fear and decreases the professional's tendencies to try to appear omnipotent, a major barrier in establishing healthy family-provider relationships.

Train to take the "heat" for past and present errors. Over the years, family members of the chronically ill have been exposed to many treatments that have been insensitive, ineffective, or blatantly wrong. Hopefully, these hurtful practices are decreasing in frequency; but still today, most of us are challenged to explain indefensible actions on the part of our colleagues. Try as we may to avoid it, we also continue to make mistakes ourselves, and it is likely that the next generation of mental health professionals will do the same. A major change in family-provider relationships could be facilitated if professionals could be trained to absorb the legitimate criticisms of family members and to handle them without becoming defensive. Most of the family members of chronic patients that professionals of our era will encounter during their careers will have reason to be angry and frustrated, even if this particular professional is attempting to be "different." Changed practices and changed relationships will only be possible if newly trained professionals can learn to take the blame for past and present mistakes and continue to listen and be available even when they feel unappreciated. They must then be trained to use this feedback from families, along with their own influence, to lobby for modified practices. This means that training professionals to work differently with families will require, for the foreseeable future, that they also be trained to tolerate the stress of being an intermediary between families, other health-care professionals, and larger systems. Interdisciplinary cooperation is not easy under any circumstances, and the acceptance of what was originally termed the "ombudsman role" with families (Anderson et al. 1980) adds incredible stress to the professional who must perform these functions. This role means absorbing everyone's requests and everyone's anger, while never giving up the attempt to be a bridge, a way for each component of a system to understand the other. Special support networks must be established to enable professionals to continue in this role over time.

Emphasize basic assumptions in training.   The skills we provide to professionals are, as Dr. Bernheim suggested, crucial. However, I believe we must also include explicit attention to a few basic assumptions that too often go unexamined. Some I have already mentioned: 1) there is honor and reward in devoting a lifelong career to the chronically ill; 2) information can produce change; and 3) families and professionals can, and should, find more productive ways of collaborating. I would like to emphasize one more: the importance of assuming a nonjudgmental stand with families and making the assumption of "least pathology" until proven otherwise (Pinsof 1983).

Most of the professional training in all health-related disciplines is focused on identifying pathology. We are taught to pursue and describe the unusual, the negative, the things that do not work well. Unless a specific effort is made to challenge and contradict this tendency, professionals will look at families in this same way. Unfortunately, this perspective is not only not the most helpful one, but it can do actual damage. All families have problems, and all families have strengths. We must learn to look at and respect both, without assuming that all families with a chronically ill member are pathological. Some may be, some may not be. Learning to interact with families while making an assumption of least pathology, however, should not be equated with an assumption that the needs of families of chronic patients should not be addressed unless they are pathological. Rather, I would suggest that all families, however strong, have certain needs for support and information in times of a crisis or stress of this sort. Some families will have the need for more help because they experience multiple stresses, some perhaps totally unrelated to the patient's illness. Some families will have ways of relating that would be problematic under any circumstances and are even more so considering the specific issues presented by a chronic illness. In other words, the provision of or need for services to families, therefore, should not be equated with an assumption of pathology on the family's part. No one, including family members, should be required to accept a definition of "pathological" in order to be offered or to accept help in coping with something as devastating as a mental illness.

Implant a healthy skepticism. Although we are learning more every day, we know very little about these devastating illnesses. Unfortunately, many professionals tend to become wedded to the particular theories and therapies they were exposed to in their training, whether or not there is evidence for their effectiveness. Our educational programs do not go far enough in teaching professionals to evaluate data, literature, and experiences in a critical manner. Too often, decisions are made on the basis of belief systems that have not been reevaluated in the light of new knowledge. The inculcation of an attitude of healthy skepticism in evaluating the current state of the art and the limits of new findings is vital to the long-term development of more rational treatment programs and a more balanced relationship between families and service providers on an ongoing basis.

SUMMARY

Despite the best intentions of families and professionals to establish and maintain new, more productive, more collaborative relationships, there are systems issues that can mitigate against this process over time. First, administrators of some mental health systems are often reluctant to involve families in the care of patients and are reluctant to provide the staff and facilities that would make this possible. In some cases, it is because they see families as irrelevant to patient care. In some cases, it is because families do not fit easily into hospital procedures and it is "inconvenient" to include their opinions and needs. In other cases, there is a definite fear of families, who are seen as angry, unreasonable, and potentially threatening to the administration's control of their own services. They worry that if families get active or learn too much, health systems will have to become accountable. In my view, this would be a healthy outcome but I do believe we must prepare our trainees (and ourselves) for ongoing resistance to change in this arena.

Second, many administrators of health care systems do not welcome programs for families, particularly those designed to help family members keep patients out of hospitals. There is no financial incentive to provide outpatient treatment, and usually no financial reimbursement for educational workshops for relatives. Training programs that address these issues may also find themselves out of favor when the funds for research or demonstration projects are eliminated. The economics of health care can be more powerful than clinical judgment or perceived family need in determining which programs survive.

Finally, we must, in our training, emphasize the need for continuity of services over time. Surviving in the face of chronic illness requires an ongoing relationship between families, patients, and health care providers, not a crisis-oriented program. Several of the new models of patient care that involve families appear to be at least somewhat more effective than others that have been attempted in the past (for example, Hogarty et al. 1986; Falloon et al. 1982; Leff et al. 1982). None of these programs simply give families information about schizophrenia. Yet, second-generation programs are developing that do little more than describe the illness and tell relatives to tone down the intensity of family life. This type of education is probably not enough to help anyone to cope with a devastating mental illness and its ramifications on an ongoing basis. For most patients and their families, the illness will require at least intermittent attention for many years. Because disruptions in the relationship with treatment systems are extremely upsetting for patients, and thus ultimately for families, programs offering only brief educational interventions without consistent follow-up may not be truly helpful. In fact, they may even add to the problems and frustrations faced by patients and families by implying that there is an "easy" recipe for successful management of chronic mental illness, without offering to help to implement it.

I believe, therefore, that despite current tendencies to reject family interventions, professionals should be trained to provide them. I would rather see us change what is called treatment than eliminate it. I am concerned that the current righteous anger over attitudes toward and treatment of families of patients with mental illness will cause reasonable, vital, and useful treatment programs to be rejected along with those that are indefensible. I know that some relatives' organizations are currently taking a stand that rejects all psychosocial research and all family treatment. If this policy were to be adopted, I believe the result could be even fewer services to patient's families and less respect for what it means to provide for these patients in their homes and in their communities. Biological research is vital. However, even if major advances occur in understanding brain structure and chemistry, those who have a mental illness today or who develop one in the next 10–20 years will not reap many of the benefits. Someone should still be available who knows how to help patients live with their illnesses and how to help families live with patients.

A few short years ago, deinstitutionalization was touted as a major solution to the problems of mental illness. The problems of patients, we were told, were caused by unnecessary hospitalization, and the "right to refuse treatment" and "informed consent" became battle cries. However, as Phyllis Vine (1982) stated:

> The just and human spirit which today prevents one relative from placing another in an uncaring hospital where many people wasted thirty years ago also provides little comfort for a mother who sees her daughter slowly starving to death, a man who sees his brother aimlessly wandering and taking refuge on a bus bench, or a child who watches a parent isolate himself to the point of nonexistence.

These problems and the pain they engender are not going to go away. The discovery of a new neurotransmitter or increased understanding of structural variations in the brain through PET scans will be of small comfort to the family who needs to know how to cope with their son's delusions or how to help their daughter to do more than sleep or to find a way to make some sort of place for herself in an unresponsive world.

REFERENCES

Anderson CM, Hogarty GE, Reiss DJ: Family treatment of adult schizophrenic patients: a psychoeducational approach. Schizophr Bull 6:490–505, 1980

Anderson CM, Reiss DJ, Hogarty GE: Schizophrenia and the Family. New York, Guilford, 1986

Falloon I, Boyd JS, McGill CW, et al: Family management in the prevention of exacerbations of schizophrenia. N Engl J Med 306:1437–1440, 1982

Hogarty GE, Anderson CM, Reiss DJ, et al: Family psycho-education, social skills training and maintenance: chemotherapy in the aftercare treatment of schizophrenia. Arch Gen Psychiatry 43:633–642, 1986

Leff J, Kuipers L, Berkowitz R, et al: A controlled trial of social intervention in the families of schizophrenia patients. Br J Psychiatry 141:121–134, 1982

Pinsof W: Integrative problem-solving therapy: toward the synthesis of family and individual psychotherapies. Journal of Marital and Family Therapy 9:19–36, 1983

Vine P: Families in Pain. New York, Pantheon, 1982

Chapter 5

Research Directions for a New Conceptualization of Families

Harriet P. Lefley, Ph.D.

Behavioral research on families and mental illness for the most part has focused on etiology—on assumptions regarding the family's role in generating, precipitating, or exacerbating psychotic disorder in the patient. Studies have dealt primarily with hypothesized characteristics and interactional patterns and, in more recent prospective studies, with the predictive power of antecedent relationships and conditions. For the most part, research has centered on the schizophrenias. For this reason, it is difficult to discuss theoretical and empirical issues in the literature without restricting the discussion to one set of disorders, although it is believed that clinicians' beliefs, attitudes, and behavior toward families generalize across diagnostic categories.

In contrast to the above emphasis, most of the chapters in this book focus on the experiential impact of mental illness on the family, including the interrelated consequences of theorizing, training emphases, treatment approaches, service delivery models, and social policy. The book focuses particularly on the sequelae of common theoretical paradigms—on the behaviors and policies that flow from certain conceptual models of family-patient relationships and from their correlative modes of family-clinician interaction. This combined impact on the family has a great deal to do with the nature and extent of participation of the patient's relatives in the treatment process.

The impact of mental illness on significant others has typically been subsumed under the heading of objective and subjective family

burden (Platt 1985). Family burden is only now coming to the fore
as a significant social problem because of increasing numbers of patients with Alzheimer's disease. The traumatizing aspects of living with
severe mental illness, however, have received relatively little attention
in the literature as a research issue, in contrast to the deviant role
relationships and disordered communication patterns that have been
the focus of the majority of studies (Liem 1980). This is rather surprising because, in many respects, behaviors of patients with Alzheimer's disease and those designated as functionally psychotic are
similar, e.g., bizarre behaviors, cognitive deficit, paranoia, and deterioration from a previous level of functioning. Additionally, as Wasow
(1985) has suggested, there may be even greater pain in the loss of
persons who typically represent one's future rather than one's past.
The few empirical studies that have been done on family burden in
dealing with psychotic disorders uniformly indicate a high degree of
emotional and financial distress among wives of hospitalized patients
(Clausen and Yarrow 1955), parents of psychotic children (Arey and
Warheit 1980), children of mentally ill parents (Grunebaum et al.
1982; Keller et al. 1986), and families of deinstitutionalized adult
patients (Doll 1976; Hatfield 1978; Herz et al. 1976; Lefley 1987a;
Noh and Turner 1987). There is little evidence, however, that this
reactive emotional distress has been viewed as a legitimate concern
worthy of the attention of mental health professionals, beyond its
relationship to the care of the identified patient.

Family burden is just one of many issues, however. Increasing
attention to treatment outcome with the long-term, severe mental
illnesses, particularly the schizophrenias, has indicated two phenom-
ena of concern to families: 1) Despite years of treatment by a wide
range of therapists in the system, a substantial number of patients
remain chronically impaired (Gardos et al. 1982; McGlashan 1984).
2) Except for chemotherapy, the major therapies that clinicians have
been trained to administer are not perceived as sufficiently beneficial
by significant others who have observed the patient over the years
(Hatfield 1983b; Holden and Lewine 1982; Lefley 1987c).

It is the latter finding that is critical for clinical education. Families
of the severely impaired mentally ill do not give high ratings to individual or family therapy for themselves or for their loved ones.
Moreover, it is empirically evident that many patients whose families
have invested in years of verbal therapies are not able to attain adequate levels of functioning. This is not to say that such therapies do
not help; but they do not appear to have helped enough, given the
investment of time, money, emotional commitment, and expectancy.
Current trends in individual therapy for schizophrenic patients have
veered from a psychodynamic to a supportive focus, trying to help

the patient manage the psychological consequences of the disorder (Coursey 1989; Ruocchio 1989).

There are two other relatively recent developments that seem more responsive to patients' and families' needs: 1) psychosocial rehabilitation (Farkas and Anthony 1989; Liberman 1987), which emphasizes ego repair through competency building rather than through intrapsychic explorations, and 2) psychoeducational interventions (Anderson et al. 1986; Falloon et al. 1984), which are responsive to families' demands for information and behavior management techniques. All of these modalities require more extensive research in a number of areas, including specificity for diagnostic groups, ongoing cost-benefit comparisons with other therapeutic approaches, and implications for clinical training and social policy.

This chapter begins with some unexplored or unresolved research issues relating to implied family pathogenesis, including stressful life events in families of the mentally ill, iatrogenic effects of clinician-family interactions, and a new look at the issue of family deviance. The second section deals with the need for a sociocultural overview of research and therapy trends involving families of the mentally ill, including recommended directions for cross-cultural comparisons. Analyses of social policy implications of deinstitutionalization and associated aftercare treatment modalities involving families are suggested. This section also looks at research needed to resolve ethical and legal complexities of some theory-bound therapeutic approaches to families. The final set of topics involves new types of research that might facilitate a paradigm shift in conceptualization of families and family role. The suggested focus is on coping strengths of families and on the most appropriate roles for families in helping develop a more effective service delivery system for the long-term mentally ill.

STRESSFUL LIFE EVENTS RESEARCH

Despite a growing literature on life events and their psychological impact, the issue of stressful life events in families of the mentally ill has received scant attention. Overviews of research indicate that adverse life events may bring about chronic psychological distress (Thoits 1983) and, conversely, that continuing or chronic role-related stresses may exacerbate the effects of life events (Brown and Harris 1978; Pearlin et al. 1981). In their overview of the literature, however, Kessler et al. (1985) pointed out that "research on the relation between chronic stress and emotional disorder is much less developed than work on life events" (p. 538).

In this connection, the distinction between normative life transitions and catastrophic life events is highly germane (Figley and McCubbin 1983; McCubbin and Figley 1983). Instruments such as that of Holmes and Rahe (1967), which weights the effects of events that occur in the lives of most individuals, are inappropriate measures of stress among persons who live with chronic conditions, and particularly those involving periodic crises.

As Angermeyer (1985) has pointed out, in the most widely used life events scales, "you will find virtually every major event conceivable in an individual's life but you will miss the fact that a close relative has become mentally ill [which is] one of the most devastating and catastrophic events that [the individual] can experience" (p. 473). There have been few instruments developed to assess the experience of chronic and periodically intolerable stress that characterizes the lives of families of the chronically mentally ill, particularly the variable of subjective burden (Platt 1985). As detailed elsewhere (Lefley 1987a), all the stressors that typically accompany any chronic condition are present in mental illnesses, but additionally, there are ongoing interactions with crisis emergency services, the police, and a wide range of service providers who may themselves be a source of frustration and resentment. Added to this are behaviors of the patient that may elicit fear, anxiety, anger, embarrassment, sadness, grieving, or depression in the family members. A study of the experiences of 84 seasoned mental health professionals with severely mentally ill relatives suggested that stressors are substantively different from those encountered by most families. For example, in an average 1-year period, 75% of the sample reported emergency calls to the psychiatrist or primary therapist, with 50% reporting three or more calls. Over 73% had needed to hospitalize their mentally ill family member at least once during the year (patients had a life mean of 7.4 hospitalizations). Almost 51% reported calling the police at least once, and 38% had to obtain a court order for involuntary commitment at least once (Lefley 1987c). It may be assumed that in families without the professional resources available to this sample, calls to the police and ex parte orders may have been even more frequent; hypotheses about other uses of the system may, of course, go either way. In any event, the behaviors necessitating such disturbing actions have rarely been explored under the rubric of stressful life events. Certainly the nature, severity, and subjective appraisal of such events is an area that should be studied, as a preliminary to assessing the coping strategies developed by families to deal with them.

Differential impact as a function of family relationship is another area that has been inadequately studied. The systems perspective views the family as an entity in process without considering the specific problems inherent in being the sibling, child, elderly parent, or spouse of someone who is severely mentally ill, and how this affects relations with the world outside the family. Although these role relationships have been studied separately in a few studies, the research is very sparse and lacks integration. Anthony's (1970) early work on discrete life-situational strains and impact on father-husband, mother-wife, and child-sibling provided a model that unfortunately has had little therapeutic follow-up. The contemporary World Health Organization Collaborative Study on Strategies for Extending Mental Health Care indicates that in developing countries, the social burden of mental illness on the family may be severe, particularly in urban areas (Giel et al. 1983). Factors influencing the functioning of the family unit were its level of subsistence, composition, housing conditions, and developmental stage in the family life cycle. A critical variable appeared to be the family role of the afflicted individual, which could affect the socioeconomic prospects of the family as a whole and alter the life goals and expectancies of other family members. Such sequelae and changes in family structure as a result of the mental illness of a key family member (see Kreisman and Joy 1974) are understudied areas in family burden literature.

An additional source of stress is the uneven course and tempo of psychotic illnesses, and the expectancies evoked during periods of remission. If the patient is in psychotherapy at the time, remissions may be attributed to the skills of the therapist. If decompensation occurs, there is an additional source of stress and anger on both sides: disappointment of the family and possible generalization of anger to all therapists as betrayers of hope and, in many cases, displaced anger of the frustrated therapist on the "sabotaging" family.

CLINICIANS' BELIEFS AND ATTITUDES: IATROGENIC EFFECTS

In the schematic model of stressors impinging on families of the mentally ill (Figure 1), clinicians' behavior is viewed as an important variable. Iatrogenic damage may be manifested in at least four modalities: psychologically disturbing sequelae of avoidant or recriminative responses to familial overtures, as double-binding messages, as a mode of intervention whose consequences may be harmful to the patient, and as a self-fulfilling prophecy that stimulates particular types of behavior in family-provider interactions. The latter mode is part of the discussion of inferred deviance in families of schizophrenic patients and elsewhere has been discussed by Terkelsen (1983).

Iatrogenic Damage to Family Members

We know that many professionals are a priori angry at family members perceived as generating the psychosis. Family members report experiences ranging from passive-aggressive behavior (overt indifference, unnecessary evasiveness, failure to return calls or keep appointments) to open hostility. Some professionals are literally unable to suppress their need to accuse, selecting words intended to evoke punishing guilt in the offending family member. A former president of a state chapter of the National Alliance for the Mentally Ill (NAMI) recounts an interaction that caused her intense and long-lasting pain:

> Some years ago, when my oldest son became ill with schizophrenia, my husband and I drove 200 miles to the state hospital where he had been committed. I can't describe to you my anguish and horror at seeing my child hospitalized. We met with the hospital superintendent, a psychiatrist, and I said, "Doctor, we love our son dearly and want to do everything possible to help him recover. Please tell us what we can do."
> The doctor responded contemptuously, "I think you have already done quite enough, mother."
> "What do you mean?" I cried.
> "After all," he said coldly, "it was in your home that he became ill."

Iatrogenic Damage to Patients

Family theories may create undue problems for the so-called identified patient, while adding to the distress of already overburdened family members. The following true case history illustrates the way in which an inappropriate intervention may begin to systematically destroy a patient's support system.

A young wife and mother of two small children describes her life situation for the past 2 years with her schizophrenic husband:

> My husband Bill had lost his second job in a year and started falling apart. He couldn't work so I had to find a job, find babysitters, and take over full care of the family. Bill started getting more and more delusional, and life was a living hell for me and the children. Finally, Bill got so psychotic that he had to be taken to Crisis, and then he was sent up to the state hospital.
> After working all week at a very demanding job, every Sunday I get up real early, find a different babysitter—which isn't easy on a Sunday—and then take a 2-hour bus ride to visit Bill. He usually doesn't talk much. But for the last 3 months he's been having psychotherapy with a young psychologist who's doing his internship there. Bill has started saying mean things to me, like "You know,

you've gotten to be very controlling"—as if I don't have to control things now!—and "My shrink thinks you have a need for me to be sick. He thinks you get something out of my symptoms."

I don't know what to do except cry. For the first time, I started thinking, "What *do* I need this for? If I stay with him, my life will go down the drain."

One wonders about the rationale for the treatment plan in cases like this, about the quality of supervision, and about the very real problem of psychological damage to someone who has every right to expect appreciation and instead receives recrimination. These indictments, filtered through a psychotic husband without benefit of marital therapy, can only stretch an already overburdened and bewildered wife to the breaking point. The words will also embed themselves in her consciousness, because whether the couple stays together or separates, the wife will undoubtedly feel the guilt that our culture teaches families to feel in cases of mental illness. In this case, of course, responsibility for her husband's illness has received the professional imprimatur. Most importantly, this type of naive "therapy" can only serve to erode a family system already severely stressed by the reality demands of the husband's illness.

The educational aspects of this case are self-evident. First is the need for therapists to understand the existential impact of mental illness on a spouse in a two-parent nuclear family (see Anthony 1970). When the therapist analyzes the marriage from the patient's recounting of their life together, how is "controlling" and intrusive behavior interpreted in a woman who has had to take over all the affairs of the family and protect her children from harm? Second is the clinician's need to understand the effects of his or her interpretations, i.e., to recognize that antagonism may be evoked by exposing dependency needs in any husband, but particularly in one who is too impaired to control his rage at his own inadequacies as husband and father.

To understand how such therapy may ultimately prove detrimental to the patient, the clinician must understand the situation within a paradigm of stress, coping, and adaptation, rather than one of pathogenesis (Hatfield and Lefley 1987). Otherwise, therapists may contribute to the very systems breakdown they are trying to prevent. The development of such educational models, and their testing as clinical tools, is an important aim.

The Iatrogenic Double Bind

Another important stressor involves the cognitive dissonance evoked by conflicting messages from mental health professionals. The confusion engendered in dealing with multiple psychiatrists of differing persuasions and treatment approaches has been outlined in numerous books, most cogently by Wechsler et al. (1988). Thurer (1983), claiming deinstitutionalization is essentially a women's issue, depicts the following mental health risks for the overburdened care giver, typically the mother: 1) suffering from the pain of sickness in her child; 2) suffering from the stigmatization of having "caused the illness"; 3) overseeing a treatment plan that may be unrealistic in terms of time, energy, money, and the demands of the rest of the family; and 4) receiving conflicting advice from various professionals with little promise of success. "When things do not go smoothly, she is blamed. Should she discourage her child from unnecessary risks, she may be deemed overprotective. Should she encourage independence and seek residential placement, she may be deemed neglectful or rejecting. Should she demur from following any professional advice, she may be called a 'saboteur' " (p. 1163). Moreover, as Thurer noted, in the contemporary climate this care giver is not even applauded for self-sacrifice when she cannot fulfill the expectancies of a liberated woman.

Family members who wish to educate themselves about mental illness may also receive contradictory messages from the literature. On the one hand is a "prevention" literature that teaches symptom recognition and urges earliest possible psychiatric intervention. On the other hand are books and articles issuing caveats about the dangers of labeling, the perils of hospitalization, and possible adverse effects of neuroleptics. The variable benefits of different types of psychotherapy are, of course, a constant issue (see Klerman 1984; Torrey 1988). Family consumers are thus faced with a literature that urges the use of a system that an equally reputable literature tells them is fraught with perils for the patient.

For those who have been exposed to different schools of family therapy, there may be an implicit double bind in the technologies used. Many theoretical models are subsumed under a general rubric of lack of genuineness in communication. These models suggest that in families of schizophrenic patients, people say what they do not mean and mean what they do not say (Hoffman 1981). In any textbook on family therapy, numerous examples are given of how the therapist redirects the interaction process, including issuing paradoxical injunctions, so that hidden agendas may be aired and resolved. In psychoeducational interventions, however, families are taught how to suppress affect and carefully choose their words with patients subject to undue psychophysiological arousal. Kanter (1985c) has maintained that the "benign indifference" suggested by Anderson et al. (1986) as a mode of refraining from criticism is impossible to sustain among clinicians, let alone relatives in constant contact with the patient. These may indeed be confusing issues for family members eager to learn the most appropriate behavior management techniques.

McFarlane and Beels (1983) have suggested an implicit double bind in the dual messages conveyed to families by basically disapproving clinicians. "If one accepts that double-bind interactions can create distorted, even irrational, communication, then many 'therapeutic' situations can be seen as pathogenic: For instance, covert blame of the family by professionals is often combined with overt attempts to help them, while the contradiction is denied" (p. 316).

Above all, the double bind may emanate from the basic armature of many schools of family therapy that emphasize authenticity while failing to deal authentically or even using subterfuge with patients. Maranhao (1984) has sharply criticized systems therapy on this head: "If therapists are willing . . . to hide pieces of information in order to lead their interlocutors to certain beliefs, and if they are ready to say and do things they do not believe, then they must consider these attributes acceptable when displayed in family life" (p. 277).

Research Issues

The personal anecdotes recounted earlier are critical to any thesis of iatrogenic damage. They raise several important research issues, presented here as sequential, interrelated areas of investigation.

Frequency of negative interactions. The small body of literature on interactions of families of the mentally ill with clinicians treating their relatives suggests that negative experiences are not uncommon (Appleton 1974; Group for the Advancement of Psychiatry 1986; Hatfield 1978; Holden and Lewine 1982; Lamb 1983). An ancillary literature suggests that depreciating attitudes may also be found in professionals' interactions with families of autistic children (Culbertson 1977) and even with families of the mentally retarded (Turnbull and Turnbull 1978). More systematic research is needed to determine whether this type of behavior is indeed an unacknowledged problem affecting significant numbers of consumers.

Impact on family members. Does the type of behavior described in the preceding anecdotes constitute a risk factor for emotional distress or decompensation among 1) individuals already suffering from massive situational stressors and/or 2) a group of persons of whom a subset may be unusually vulnerable to subclinical or spectrum disorders? To date, we have a descriptive literature that speaks of "iatrogenic anguish" (Bernheim and Lehman 1985, p. 10) but no hard data on the extent to which family members have been adversely affected. This is a related but separate issue from the dissatisfactions with mental health services reported by Hatfield (1978) and Holden and Lewine (1982), because it postulates an actively harmful role on the part of some clinicians.

Several research models may lend themselves to investigation of some of these hypotheses. A multiple-regression formula determining whether specific types of theoretical beliefs may predict interactional patterns is warranted. Although attitudes may be masked in the well-trained clinician, there are sufficient indications in the literature to suggest that family members can perceive devaluing messages. Operational questions are 1) Do interactions with particular types of therapists result in diminished self-esteem, anger, feelings of humiliation, or other emotionally distressing reactions on the part of family members? 2) Are adverse familial reactions reflected directly or indirectly in adverse impact on the patient?

Defensive strategies.   The cases described previously suggest the possibility that threats to ego strength or coping capabilities of family members may weaken a system already buffeted by situational stressors. This is a critically important hypothesis, involving some corollary questions. What are the defensive strategies used by family members? Does the family member's history of experiences with providers—which may span many years—generate expectancies of evasiveness, dissembling, deflection of questions, or attitudinal rejection? Do these expectancies in turn produce anticipatory aggressive, demanding, or even threatening behavior in order to receive answers or services? Or alternatively, does the expected rejection reinforce a tendency to become overly submissive and compliant or withdraw from confrontation and accelerate the process of disengagement or even abandonment of the patient? Is there a predictable pattern of familial behaviors that are perceived as adverse by mental health professionals? Are these behaviors in turn related to the patient's length of stay in the provider system, and to the number and types of familial interactions with professionals?

Attitudinal antecedents.   To what extent are adversarial attitudes in mental health professionals a predictable product of clinical training, beginning with basic undergraduate education in the social sciences? There are many impressionistic observations that our basic texts on social and clinical issues have emphasized an adverse family role in the development of all emotional and mental disorders. Even when these theories are embedded in a framework of multiple etiologies, the sheer numbers of references to family pathology are believed to result both in quantitative and qualitative emphases on bad parenting as a major antecedent. An analysis of mother blaming in 125 articles in major clinical journals for a 3-year period found 72 different types of psychopathology attributed to mothers (Caplan and Hall-McCorquodale 1985a), with little change over time. These authors and others have called for a halt in the scapegoating of mothers by professionals (Caplan and Hall-McCorquodale 1985b; Chess 1982).

There are numerous hypotheses here that merit testing. 1) In any probability sample of mental health professionals, regardless of discipline, a significant number will be willing to make a priori generalizations about parents of mentally ill patients without a case history. For example, if faced with a stimulus of "mother of a child with schizophrenia" versus "mother of a child with leukemia," the respondent will make significantly more negative attributions about the motivations and behavior of the former without any further information. 2) If the reference point is the raters' feelings about the stimulus figures, they will be significantly less sympathetic toward the parents of the schizophrenic child. 3) Biologically oriented professionals will show significantly less disparity in their ratings than their behaviorally oriented peers. 4) Students given various etiological theories to read, counterbalanced for biogenic versus psychogenic models, would show significant differences in their treatment of a role-playing "parent of a schizophrenic." The perception by the person doing the role-playing of the efficacy and understanding of the interviewing student would similarly vary as a function of the interviewer's theories.

We could go on and on with these types of paradigms, but the inference is clear. It is anticipated that without any type of case contextualization, parents of psychotic patients will be seen as unattractive and possibly destructive personalities, less able to feel compassion than parents of children with other disorders. As a corollary, it is hypothesized that clinicians will have significantly more negative personal feelings toward the former group. The second area of study would then pertain to parental perceptions of and reactions to these events. How does the "negatively valued other" respond to disapprobation, particularly when this is perceived as emanating from the only people who can help one's sick child?

Attribution Theory

Attribution theory looks at the basic determinants of the process of causal inference. This more advanced area of research may be necessary to address the entire issue of attribution of blame, in order to deal with this process in the course of transmitting theory in clinical education. In Shaver's (1985) work in this area, assignment of blame includes concepts of causality, responsibility, and blameworthiness (presence or absence of mitigating factors). Responsibility involves levels of foreseeability and intentionality, variables that family theoreticians claim they do not attribute to families. Blameworthiness is similarly eschewed, particularly by those who believe in the "third-generation" transmission of the schizophrenias. Yet, causality is considered epistemologically unacceptable as a construct (Dell 1980). The question remains as to how negative attributions regarding the characteristics and behaviors of families develop in students and clinicians when the theories underlying their work purport to eschew the basic components of these attributions. This is a fertile area for social psychological research.

ESSENTIAL QUESTION OF FAMILY DEVIANCE

A conceptualization of families that began with pathogenesis has become truncated to the more modest hypothesis of deviation from some unformulated norm. Within the deviation framework, etiological concerns have become reduced to avoidance of familial behaviors that may exacerbate psychotic symptoms. In an otherwise excellent article, Hirsch (1979) gave an early manifestation of the ambivalence that continues to characterize the work of many who have reconstructed their attitudes toward families and family role: "There is as yet no evidence to support the view that parents bring about, in the formative years, the tendency for their children to become schizophrenic in later life" (p. 52). Yet in the same article, on the same page, discussing the work of Lidz and others, he stated, "Yet, the observations of the original observers, who were astute and experienced clinicians, have struck a note of acknowledgment in any of us who deal with schizophrenics and their parents." This notion of family deviance is still found passim in much of the psychoeducational literature.

One reason the field has begun to abjure references to familial etiology is that the related research has failed to meet the basic methodological criteria required for demonstrating the validity of the concept (Howells and Guirguis 1985; Parker 1982; Reiss 1976; Stone 1978; Terkelsen and Cole 1985). Similarly, at least two basic research criteria must be satisfied to confirm any hypothesis of deviance. The first is that of panhuman universality. Can it be demonstrated, cross-culturally and with cross-sectional (synchronic) and longitudinal (diachronic) reliability, that there is an observable pattern of deviation from culturally normative behavior in families of schizophrenic patients? The second criterion is that of frequency. Even if deviant patterns are consistently found, is deviance found in such a small subset of the universe of families with schizophrenic members that it has little relevance for science and treatment? Is it likely that the statements made about such families are based on such marginally significant differences that the findings may be attributed more parsimoniously to the common genetic link rather than to any etiologically relevant behavioral dispositions?

These questions of course have been posed before, but primarily as alternative explanations, rarely as direct targets for research. The reason they are being raised again is that the literature continues to abound with global generalizations about the characteristics of families of schizophrenic patients as if these were modal or normative for this population. Reynolds and Farberow (1981), for example, stated, "In addition to genetic factors there seem to be at least five characteristics attributable to schizophrenic families: 1) excessively closed family systems; 2) shared family myths or delusions; 3) paralogic modes of thinking in all the family members; 4) lack of individuation and self-identity of members from the family 'ego mass' . . .; and 5) intense, pathological symbiotic attachments of the child to parents and of parents to grandparents" (p. 126). Schuman (1983) divides families of hospitalized schizophrenic patients into just two categories: the "schizophrenic family," in which all members function at a very low level, and the "family with a schizophrenic member," in which "there may be high levels of social or vocational achievement; on an emotional level, however, significant members possess low levels of self. They function with what Bowen has described as a 'pseudo-self' rather than solid self" (Schuman 1983, p. 43). As Liem (1980) has pointed out, treatment of family characteristics has been analogous to a trait theory perspective, prompting the unwarranted generalization of relationships that may pertain for a small subgroup to all families with schizophrenic members.

An interesting notion of "normal deviance" has been suggested by Angermeyer (1985), a West German researcher who studied communication deviance in a follow-up of families of formerly hospitalized schizophrenic patients 2 years after discharge. He found that "normal" patterns were seen only in families whose schizophrenic members had required rehospitalization. On the other hand, "families with patients with a better outlook 'deviate' from the common standard norm. This suggests that the rather detached relationships (which allude to some aspects of the concept of low 'Expressed Emotion' [EE]) observed in families with patients who are not readmitted may indicate the successful adjustment to the new situation" (p. 476).

Angermeyer cited the work of Cheek (1965), who in a similar paradigm found that "apparently the more 'normal' the family on most of the characteristics which differentiate between families of 'normals' and 'schizophrenics,' the worse the outcome of the schizophrenic . . . Our study has revealed a characteristic distortion of the family environment . . . which shows up most notably in the area of social control. In the absence of certain aspects of this distortion the convalescent schizophrenic deteriorates" (p. 145). Angermeyer has concluded that interaction patterns previously considered dysfunctional "prove now to be functional, hence normal . . . I think this could help us to better tolerate previously assumed deviance and would make us hesitate more from calling families 'abnormal,' 'pathologic,' or even 'pathogenic.' This in turn might even help families to cope better with schizophrenic illness" (p. 478).

The notion that communication deviance is a salutary accommodation is in contrast to most of the literature. Moreover, communication deviance has been viewed as an antecedent more than a reactive condition (possibly genetically based). McFarlane (1983), discussing family factors correlated with schizophrenia, has suggested that "coexistence of EE and [communication deviance] may be not only specific to but predictive of schizophrenia before the initial episode" (p. 144). Assuming covariance of the two dimensions, and continuity of prodromal stages, this suggests 1) a genetic analogue or 2) a parental reactive mode that may or may not contribute to decompensation but that, in its most parsimonious interpretation, reflects an adaptation to living with difficult prepsychotic children.

Figure 1 presents a possible explanatory model for the perception of deviance in families of patients with psychotic disorders. I have not attempted to grapple here with prodromal reactive modes, nor with the distinctions in stress levels experienced by families with schizophrenic, bipolar, or other major psychotic disorders. These may be similar enough to fit into the model or may vary along specified dimensions as a function of the patient's levels of contact, functioning, and productivity; frequency of psychotic episodes; and capacity for interactional and instrumental rewards. Overall, regardless of diagnostic category, I believe that "deviant" behavior may well be the generalized product of the multiply determined stressors previously discussed and indicated in Figure 1. Moreover, those elements of familial deviance manifested as anger, assertiveness, resistance, or sabotage may in fact be adaptive responses to a therapeutic field of confusion, contradiction, and multiple failures.

CROSS-CULTURAL ISSUES

When considering the family and mental illness in cultural context, a number of issues appear to be highly variable across cultures and warrant further investigation. These include 1) apparent differences in attitudes and conceptualization of family role on the part of

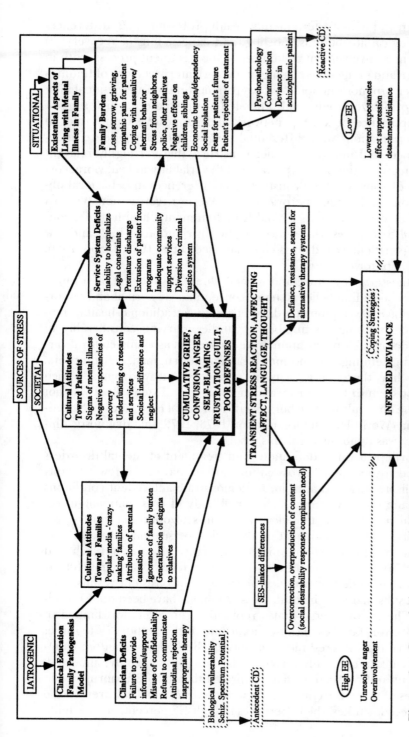

Figure 1. Cumulative stress model in families of schizophrenic patients leading to inferred deviance by mental health professionals. CD = communication deviance. EE = expressed emotion. SES = socioeconomic status.

Western and non-Western mental health professionals; 2) differences in etiological attributions, labeling, and expectations of recovery; 3) differential involvement of families in the treatment process, both in Western and indigenous healing models; 4) interpretations of findings of better prognosis in non-Western patients (in the International Pilot Study of Schizophrenia and other follow-up studies), which suggest the importance of kinship network and supportive family role; 5) value orientations with differential weighting of dependence, independence, and interdependence constructs that are highly relevant to aftercare models and expectancies; 6) variability in behavioral correlates of some of these constructs; 7) differences in behavioral observations and diagnostic practices of Western versus non-Western and United States versus United Kingdom mental health professionals; and 8) manifest differences in the distribution of high and low EE cross-nationally and cross-culturally (see Lefley 1984, 1985b, 1986, and 1987b, for citations).

The study of culture and mental illness has focused on a range of issues including belief systems, conceptions of normal and abnormal behavior, symptomatic differences, and traditional healing modalities. A substantial number of studies, varying considerably in methodological sophistication, have focused on assessing cultural variation in defining, diagnosing, treating, and stigmatizing disorders. For a while, there was a focus on "culture-bound syndromes," which did not seem to fit a universal diagnostic grid. Essentially it was not until the nine-culture collaborative International Pilot Study of Schizophrenia (World Health Organization 1973, 1979) that diagnostic uniformity was established for this disorder.

Perhaps because definitions and treatment of mental disorders have been so variable across cultures, there have been few attempts to replicate studies that claim to demonstrate antecedent conditions of a panhuman syndrome. The small body of cross-national–cross-cultural research on etiological factors in schizophrenia shows great disparity, perhaps contingent on theoretical persuasion (Alanen 1966). Efforts to replicate communication deviance research (Hirsch and Leff 1975) or to explore the construct through new paradigms (Blakar 1980) have tended to produce negative or inconsistent results. The only results that have held up cross-nationally have been the EE findings. The major United States replication, however, was limited to Anglo-Saxon families because, according to the authors (Vaughn et al. 1984), high interethnic variability in the United Kingdom counterindicated a culturally mixed replication. Subsequently, almost all cross-cultural replications have indicated that low EE is normative in families of schizophrenic persons in more traditional cultures. In the most recent studies, the differences in high-EE percentages are quite remarkable: 54% in England and Denmark versus 23% in India (Wig et al. 1987); in California, 67% in Anglo-American versus 41% in Mexican American samples (Jenkins et al. 1986). In an American inner-city area, the relationships between EE and relapse were sustained, but not for blacks, who comprised two-thirds of the sample (Moline et al. 1985). EE continues to be a critical area for cross-cultural research.

Another issue of particular interest is cultural variation in the self-perception of families and their related responses in both clinical and research settings. Is there an anticipatory effect as a function of sophistication in Western etiological theory? Most families in the Western world are exposed to popular media articles on child rearing and assumptions of parental culpability when children are emotionally disabled. Do these theories generate varieties of intrapunitive behavior that include fulfilling perceived negative expectancies of clinicians or researchers? Is there more guilt among the better-educated? A number of studies have shown that group differences in communication deviance findings were significant only for subjects higher on the socioeconomic scale (Liem 1980), suggesting an intragroup response style that may indeed be an artifact of subcultural differences. Response-style differences are likely to be even more pronounced in comparisons of Western subjects with counterparts who have no knowledge of presumed family role.

The impact of value orientations on theory is of particular importance. It is paradoxical that anthropologically derived theories such as Haley's (1980) should be so ethnocentric in their central postulates and applications. The assumption that young adults must leave home as a normal process, and that they remain only to hold warring parents together, is quintessentially culture bound. It is based on Western family structure and life-styles, and on Western notions of independence involving physical separation from the family of origin. It is by now axiomatic that Western psychological theory has largely ignored the extended kinship or clan networks that have generated multiple significant others in child rearing: the nanny, maid, older sibling, grandmother, neighbor, and most importantly in many matrilineal cultures, the maternal uncle. It is these networks that Leff (1981) has suggested fulfill an important buffering role in the care of schizophrenic family members. The "low stress–high social support" explanatory model that Mosher and Keith (1981) have applied to the International Pilot Study of Schizophrenia findings is based in large part on the resources provided by the extended family and its ability to reintegrate the patient into a viable social role.

The Israeli High-Risk Study (Mirsky et al. 1985) has raised extremely important issues regarding the significance of the role of

parents, peers, and professional care givers in the developmental career of preschizophrenic children. Comparisons of matched groups
of kibbutz- and town-reared high-risk children showed the highest
incidence of psychiatric disorders in kibbutz index cases, reared by a
professional care giver (metapelet) rather than by a schizophrenic
parent. Explanations of the data have suggested that it is precisely
the lack of a close and protective mother-child relationship as opposed
to the "evenhanded benevolence" of the metapelet that might pre-
dispose a vulnerable child (Kety 1985). It has also been suggested that
in a cultural setting in which it is not the family but the peer group
that is "the authority and the source of constraints and standards" (p.
359), the vulnerable child may not be able to respond appropriately
in this type of high-demand situation and may escape into loneliness
(Breznitz 1985). This again highlights the need to understand the
structure of the unit involved in child rearing.

Ultimately, any generalizations about family relations and mental
illness will have to be validated on the hard crucible of cross-cultural
comparison and replication. This is based on an assumption of transcultural uniformities of biogenic disorders, with cultural variation in
definition, appraisal, acceptance, environmental stressors and supports, and correlative self-evaluation on the part of the patient. It is
precisely these variations in societal response that may yield valuable
clues to the most salutary treatment and care-giving environments for
psychotic disorders.

FAMILY ROLE AND SOCIAL POLICY

Social Implications of EE Research

As several contributors have noted, the EE literature has raised
numerous important issues relevant to family-patient relationships.
There are important policy implications in the psychoeducational interventions that comprise the major modality for applying the findings. First is the apparent assumption that the emotional interactions
of families with patients are more invested with pathogenic possibilities than those of other care givers; second is that families are the
primary care givers and therefore are more significant for training
than other categories of persons, e.g., foster-home parents, residential
managers, day-treatment workers, case managers, and psychotherapists.

The repeated statement by the EE researchers themselves that
EE is just one contextual example of psychophysiological arousal under environmental stress obviously merits continuing research into
the range and nature of toxic stimuli. Vaughn et al. (1984) stated that

"it is for other researchers to explain the considerable relapse rates (even when receiving optimal drug therapy) of schizophrenic patients who do not live with families" (p. 1177). They suggested looking to the postdischarge environment to contain at least some of the answers.

Despite the predictive value of high EE, there have been critics of the concept of low EE as a preferred alternative. Hatfield et al. (1987) suggested that suppression of affect may have adverse effects on family members and may even lead to apathy and withdrawal. Kanter (1985a) stated that relatives low in EE "express helplessness . . . While these families appear more receptive to professional input, they are often reluctant to establish firm expectations and are subject to ongoing exploitation" (p. 25). An even more important issue is the implication that patients' decompensation is most often caused by external influences over which they have no control. Kanter (1985b) has commented that family-etiology theories have absolved patients of responsibility for their actions, and with psychoeducational interventions aimed at curbing excessive stimuli, "the moral content of disturbing behavior is ignored" (p. 55). The notion of familial responsibility for the patient's behavior is one that removes control from the patient. Therapy based on this premise may reinforce infantilization by failing to respect the patient's own capabilities for averting incipient psychosis (Breier and Strauss 1983).

Family Role in Deinstitutionalization

Some years ago, Arnoff (1975) predicted deleterious social consequences for families as a result of social policies accelerating deinstitutionalization. Although families for the most part have supported community alternatives to hospitalization, the insufficiency of community support services and diminishing federal and state funding have necessitated a more active role for the private and volunteer sectors in resource development. This has raised the issue of family responsibility for providing housing for deinstitutionalized patients and supplementing the provider system with resources and volunteer services.

Social role issues: age, socioeconomic status, and gender. NAMI has generally taken the position that families must not be considered primary care givers and providers of housing. Former president James Howe (1985) has delineated the enormous tensions in caring for a mentally ill family member, including the heavy toll on well children living at home. Apart from the patient's difficulty in attaining independence in the parental home, the major issue is that residential care giving to adult children is not an appropriate role for aging parents at a time in life when they have the least energy to invest in this type of emotionally and physically draining effort. This demand may be an unrecognized mental health risk for older persons (Lefley 1987a). A related area of social policy involves family role in the provider system. Limited resources, exclusionary policies, and selective admission criteria of many community mental health programs have necessitated development of alternative services and even residential facilities by family groups.

This participation in service provision involves very serious issues of public policy—namely, the role of government and locus of responsibility for care of the disabled. In the case of the mentally ill, the issue is compounded by the fact that a disproportionate number of severely disabled patients are from lower socioeconomic strata (Dohrenwend et al. 1980). These are the patients whose families are least likely to be able to afford or develop community alternatives. An emphasis on families providing for their own relatives or even their own communities may accelerate an already emergent two-tier system of care.

Primary care giving and service provision appear to be largely performed by women. Surveys of families of the mentally ill indicate that women comprise the majority of respondents (Ascher-Svanum and Sobel 1989; Lefley 1987a), are the majority of those who join advocacy organizations (Spaniol et al. 1984), and are most likely to be care givers for deinstitutionalized patients (Thompson and Doll 1982). Thurer (1983) has pointed out that because women have traditionally been and continue to be primary care givers for the disabled, deinstitutionalization is very much a women's issue. This is particularly the case when home care of a disabled relative precludes seeking a career outside the home or fulfilling a vocational role for which one has been trained.

Legal complexities.   Other vital issues involve the interrelations of patients, families, and legal advocates. State laws restricting police interventions, difficulties in obtaining involuntary commitment of decompensating self-neglecting relatives, adversarial postures required in court proceedings, and legal temporal constraints that may force premature discharge of psychotic patients are frequent stressors over which families have little control.

In attempting to protect the patient from harm, and themselves from grief and enforced guardianship, families have sometimes found themselves in conflict with other sectors of the consumer-provider nexus. I have previously mentioned the work of Breier and Strauss (1983) with respect to patient self-control through attentiveness to prodromal cues, and Kanter's (1985b) work with patients on moral accountability in their behavior. The National Institute of Mental Health Community Support Program Learning Community Conferences and other national and local meetings have provided a more open forum for working out the reciprocal rights and responsibilities of patients, families, providers, human rights advocates, and the general public. A major social policy issue is the social contract implicit in these relationships. This is based on the premise that the responsibilities of families and service providers must be counterbalanced by the responsibility of patients for participating in their own healing. It has been suggested in particular, and operationally, that individuals have a moral obligation to refrain from making decisions (such as rejection of needed medication) that may ensure their dependency and encroach on the autonomy of others.

Fertile areas of social policy research thus involve 1) the long-term impact of deinstitutionalization on the lives of families as primary and secondary care givers, 2) the most appropriate roles for families in resource development and service provision, 3) means of assuring equity for consumer and provider subgroups, 4) effects on patients and families of legal and economic constraints that may result in multiple episodes of care seeking and adversely affect patient-family relations, and 5) the long-term consequences of emphasizing the rights of patients as superordinate to their survival needs. Of particular interest are the moral and legal implications of a societal enabling process, based on patients' rights, that paradoxically may reduce their capacity for informed consent and thus deprive them of the freedom to participate fully in the social process.

ETHICAL ISSUES

At this historical juncture, there is something of a parallel between research on families and mental illness, investigations of IQ in minority groups, and other types of research that have essentially been aimed at confirming a deficit hypothesis. Although there is no intent here to equate such diverse areas of investigation, all are categorical examples of the need to consider the social consequences of research, particularly when the findings may be applied in ways that are perceived as detrimental by the subjects of the research.

Increasing attention to the protection of human subjects requires institutional review boards to consider the issue of social risk, which involves the possibility of categorical harm to the study population. Certainly, little attention has been paid to the psychological impact of family-causation theories of schizophrenia on parents, except on an observational level (Lamb 1983) or as a rare research report (Lefley 1985a, 1987c). I wonder whether those families who willingly agreed to participate in the early observational studies such as those of the Yale group were given any inkling that the research involved hypotheses regarding their own role in pathogenesis; I also wonder what type of information is given in obtaining informed consent in family research today.

Family Therapy Research

In Chapter 6 of this book, McElroy raises legal, ethical, and social policy issues that should be investigated, particularly with respect to some traditional techniques in family therapy (see also Margolin 1982). An important question has been raised as to the modes of seeking the informed consent of families to their being observed through a one-way screen. When a team approach involves multiple observers, or when student observations are a requisite of the therapist's role as trainer, the family's options for refusal become extremely limited. The clinical situation thus becomes one in which the family's rights are severely curtailed, in ways that have been explicitly outlawed in research. There is patent coercion and duress in the requirement that to receive treatment for a loved one, family members must themselves be involved in a therapeutic encounter whether they will it or not.

A substantial number of research questions flow from family therapy experiences and warrant investigation for 1) theoretical and ethical rationale; 2) prevalence; 3) reactions of family members, including assessments of satisfaction and efficacy; and 4) development of alternative approaches. These questions have arisen in the context of agencies or institutions providing a range of services to a mentally ill family member, rather than in seeking the services of private practitioners whose preferred mode of therapy may be accepted or rejected at will. Examples of some ethical and policy issues are

1. May a family member be treated as an unidentified patient when he or she does not present himself or herself as a patient or consider himself or herself to be a patient?
2. In this context, as in any therapeutic encounter, does the therapist-patient relationship require informed consent by both—a mutual acknowledgment of status and role?
3. May a provider refuse services to a patient on the grounds that the treatment requires involvement of significant others who do not wish to participate?
4. May a provider refuse services to families who are willing to participate but do not wish to be observed, on the grounds that his or her preferred mode of therapy requires observation through a one-way screen?

5. If family therapy is rejected by family members on any grounds, does an institution have the obligation to provide alternative forms of therapy to a patient who is otherwise doing well in that therapeutic milieu?

McElroy has posed the question of why families allow themselves to become involved in family therapy against their will, even when they perceive themselves as being coerced and mistreated. The answers given by some family members is that they do not want the patient to suffer, that they fear retribution. In McElroy's example, such retribution actually seemed to take place. Examples are given of extremely coercive behavior to obtain consent, i.e., refusal to provide consultation regarding a patient's illness. The prevalence and frequency of this practice is an important area of investigation.

Family therapy is a relatively new modality, and the efficacy of systems approaches for the general population is still an open question (Bernal et al. 1983). We previously have not encountered the issue of coercing an unwilling individual with intact faculties into the patient role. These are extremely serious issues that warrant study in the professional disciplines, review by ethicists and legal experts, and final resolution and consensus before they are introduced as customary and accepted practices in the training of future clinicians.

COPING STRENGTHS OF FAMILIES

At the beginning of this chapter, I criticized the research literature for its focus on family psychopathology and relative inattention to family burden. An area that has been scarcely acknowledged is that of family strengths and coping mechanisms, despite their heuristic value for the training of clinicians. Indeed, the recognition of strength in adversity becomes the basis for a reframing of theory, from a conceptual model of pathology to one of stress, coping, and adaptation (Hatfield and Lefley 1987).

Complaints about a focus on psychopathology are found in other research subject groups, most notably survivors of the holocaust. Many who endured the unspeakable horrors of concentration camps have complained volubly that the psychiatric literature has emphasized parental transmission of depression and survivor guilt to an emotionally disturbed second generation, while ignoring the adaptive strengths of those who have literally risen from the ashes to create new lives and raise healthy children. Surely the research should contain at least an equal emphasis on proactive behavior.

Areas of Health

Most families with a mentally ill child also have other children, many of them productive and well functioning. Given the typically dismal picture of the dysfunctional "schizophrenogenic" family, why have the healthy children not been studied in greater depth? Research on siblings, which has been quite limited, has focused on relative impairment and reactions to familial disorder. Samuels and Chase's (1979) study of the well siblings of schizophrenic patients showed a high level of adjustment, despite predominant guilt. In an overview of other studies of siblings, they found minimal functional impairment.

Other research on successful adaptation of children and siblings of persons with psychotic disorders suggests there is a subset of "superkids" (Kauffman et al. 1979) and of resilient adolescents (Beardslee and Podorefsky 1988) who have much to teach us about protective factors in adaptation to extreme stress within the family. Despite ongoing research on children's responses to stress (Garmezy and Rutter 1983), modes of handling psychosis is an area that is relatively untouched. Most of the research has been at the descriptive level, with "invulnerability" analyzed in terms of coping styles rather than actual mechanisms mediating the differential response to extraordinarily stressful conditions. We certainly need to know why so many "schizophrenic families" produce siblings of widely disparate levels of productivity and psychological functioning. This may include a disproportionate number of siblings and other close relatives of chronic patients who choose to become mental health professionals (Lefley 1985a, 1987c). In Chapter 7 of this book, Cohen and Terkelsen indicated that when discussion was opened with social work students, a number admitted to mental illness in their own families. With the growth of NAMI, increasing numbers of educated and highly functioning individuals have been willing to "come out of the closet" about having mentally ill relatives.

The periodic speculation that high levels of intelligence and creativity found in some relatives of schizophrenic patients may be a biogenetic correlate of the disorder is a separate area of interest. What is germane to this discussion is the investigation of strengths in the individual relatives, or in the family system itself, that permit productivity to emerge and flourish despite the massive unhappiness generated by the illness. The compensatory mechanisms selected for overcoming despair, guilt, and hidden fears regarding one's own propensities for the disorder; modes of resolving adverse attitudes toward the disturbing relative; strategies for balancing multiple familial needs; psychological strengths that enable a sibling to develop his or her own interests and career while maintaining a supportive relationship with the patient; strategies for fighting demoralization and burnout; and the maintenance of family stability under conditions of extreme stress are some examples of research foci that might profitably supplant the older emphases on why the family caused the patient's illness or what they did to maintain it.

Strategies for Patient Care

Patient recognition of prodromal cues was mentioned earlier. Herz (1984) has found that relatives can usually recognize early signs of decompensation, a finding considered extremely important for therapeutic management of the patient. Family members have learned additional techniques for helping their relatives: dealing with grandiosity or despair, adjusting a patient's self-expectancies to realistic levels, teaching skills needed for negotiating the job market or the provider and welfare systems, and the like. Family members have also discovered their own techniques for regulating their reactions to bizarre or acting-out behavior, a response mode that may subsume or expand the construct of low EE.

Although we have previously discussed some unsatisfactory attributes of low EE, this has generally been considered a salutary characteristic, if only by default. It is apparent, however, that both high and low EE are as yet inadequately understood behavioral spectra, with considerable variability across samples. At the moment, each spectrum is evaluated almost entirely in terms of its predictive power. The nonverbal and attitudinal components, personality correlates, antecedents, and modes of manifestation in the home environment remain vague. Yet there is some intuitive understanding that if low EE is manifested as calm and accepting behavior, it provides a therapeutic ambience for schizophrenic patients.

Low-EE relatives have been used as role models in psychoeducational interventions to demonstrate the behaviors used in difficult or provocative situations (Berkowitz et al. 1981). The EE research has, of course, been predicated on the assumption of equivalence of psychopathology in patient comparison groups—not well demonstrated, but an essential control for inferring that it is familial style that predicts the higher relapse rate rather than predisposing characteristics of the patients. Assuming this is the case, what are the variables that facilitate development of low EE? In the same Los Angeles milieu studied by Vaughn et al. (1984), Jenkins et al. (1986) found few critical comments and modal patterns of acceptance, calm reactions to adverse behavior, and sensitivity for the patient's feelings among Mexican American families of schizophrenic patients: "The Mexican American relatives demonstrated a great deal of tolerance, patience, and respect toward the schizophrenic family member and would seldom challenge or take exception to psychotic behaviors. Many relatives reported that confrontations with a sick family member were unwise and did little to change matters" (p. 44). Overall, the families reacted with sadness rather than anger, tolerance rather than hostility. The investigators attributed this to three major factors: 1) acceptance of schizophrenia as a legitimate illness, 2) willingness to tolerate deviant behavior, and 3) strong social and economic support networks available to family members to allow for sharing and buffering the problems. I have mentioned here, and in greater detail elsewhere (Lefley 1984, 1985b, 1987b), cultural belief systems and attitudes toward mental illness that mitigate its self-stigmatizing effects on the patient. Some of these involve a worldview that is counter to Western value orientations and to our contemporary aftercare models (e.g., externalization of locus of control, limited expectancies, and preference for interdependence rather than "independent functioning"). In the United States, it is the sharing networks that have most relevance for one of the most important coping strategies developed by families in current years—advocacy and self-help.

Advocacy and Self-help

The growth and influence of NAMI since its organizing conference in 1979 provide empirical evidence of the coping capabilities of many families of the severely impaired long-term mentally ill. Many of the pathological characteristics attributed to families clearly emerge as context bound. The phenomenal growth of the family movement invalidates generalizations about inadequacies in families of schizophrenic patients. Prior "encapsulation" rapidly disappears in the supportive environment of the mutual support group. Energies are mobilized for advocacy rather than invested in futile despair. It is difficult to reconcile notions of dysfunctional individuals manifesting confused communication styles and paralogic ideation with the image of vigorous lobbyists and successful negotiators for services. We now have a national phenomenon of families advocating for service funds to pay the salaries of some of the very professionals who have categorically questioned their functional capabilities.

Because the mentally ill have lacked a national family constituency until very recently, in contrast to the developmentally disabled, the emergence, political influence, and rapid growth of the movement at this historical juncture well merit sociological investigation. One hypothesis is that it has taken a particular conjunction of historical events to bring this about. These include the societal pressures of deinstitutionalization, the discharge of large numbers of patients to their families, needs of providers and researchers for political advocacy, and a particular stage of knowledge regarding diathesis and family burden that facilitates more enlightened professional attitudes and provides firmer ground for provider-family alliances.

Joining forces for mutual support, education, advocacy, and needed resource development is probably the most salutary mode of coping with the disaster of mental illness in the family. Anyone who has attended sharing sessions of NAMI groups has heard the repeated theme of being alone with one's seemingly insoluble problems for many years, feeling demoralized and helpless, and rather dramatically attaining a new lease on life through the self-help experience.

The NAMI experience, however, differs substantively from self-help groups that focus exclusively or primarily on sharing and support. Impressionistic observations to date suggest that ventilation, information exchange, and even professional training in behavior management techniques, although highly therapeutic, are insufficient to cement group adherence. Participation in advocacy efforts is ultimately a much more powerful therapeutic tool, because it fulfills the need for action. It is not only the clinical parameters of the support group experience but the political involvement as social change agents that seem to have given new hope and functional skills to formerly demoralized family members. It is this observation that requires further testing and that may, if confirmed, provide a new basis for therapeutic interventions with families.

NEW THERAPEUTIC MODELS

How do we refocus clinical education? We have emphasized previously the deficit model that underlies almost all professional training—the need to guide patients toward corrective behavior. The deficit arises within a nexus of human relationships in which individuals are presumed to fail each other in important ways. With respect to families of the mentally ill, clinical educators have followed their customary modes of conceptualizing human behavior and apply a symbiotic armature for the experience of mental illness. Thus, the mentally ill person is dependent on the family for precipitation and definition of the disorder, while the family is dependent on the patient because of its putative need for symptoms. Clinicians are taught to deal with the family in this mode—as an extension of the disorder, as the unidentified patients whose pathogenic functions and roles have to be altered for recovery to occur (Hoffman 1981 and many others). Despite the salutary advances of psychoeducational interventions (and being atheoretical is considered salutary in this context), they too have been informed by this basic paradigm of altering relatives' harmful behavior toward patients.

As we have made explicit throughout this book, professionals are rarely taught to view the principals in this human tragedy as separate individuals. Unless a family member seeks individual therapy specifically geared toward coping with his or her feelings about the illness, family members are involved only as adjuncts to the patient's therapy. This includes psychoeducational and family systems therapy, which, despite all theoretical paradigms, is typically experienced by the participants as anchored to and ultimately focused on the needs of that person whose identified patienthood has brought everyone together.

When we consider the overwhelming reality problems of most families with respect to providing care—dealing with patient resistance and a range of adverse behaviors, trying to access an often inadequate service delivery system, and attempting to manage profound personal pain—it is evident that such persons could use help from mental health professionals. In any needs assessment, such problems would define these family members as a high-risk group. It is difficult to believe, however, that any one of our current treatment approaches is totally appropriate to meet this constellation of needs. Psychodynamic, systems, and even psychoeducational approaches focus on interpersonal rather than reality problems. Even though the latter, more enlightened modality may teach behavior management techniques that may lighten the load, no current therapeutic modality offers a direct mechanism for solving problems at the larger systems level. This may indeed require a merger of efforts of the professional and volunteer sectors.

Professional-Family Therapeutic Alliances

Individual family members have therapeutic needs for ventilation, coping stratagems, information, support, and a range of other needs related to the illness but separate from those of the patient. Current clinical training models can meet some of these needs, although often the self-help group provides a similar and potentially more cost-effective service. I have discussed the need for patients and relatives alike to access and influence a larger system whose operations and deficiencies may have a profound impact on their lives. The long-range psychological impact of this system is, unfortunately, far greater than any found in contemporary clinical interventions. In fact, if we remove family pathogenesis and its attendant corrective psychotherapies, we leave few clinical training models beyond the useful but limited psychoeducational interventions. These may have an effect on the relatives' feelings of mastery, and even on patient relapse. They are very important training models and there is no intent here to minimize this contribution to the armamentarium of skills needed by family members. But clinical interventions do not provide housing, resocialization with peers, skill building, job training, case management, and all the related activities that are essential for patients to function outside of the parental home. With a long-overdue revival of interest in the needs of the severely impaired and chronic patient, there is a strong need for psychosocial rehabilitation training models to become an integral component of clinical training curricula (see Farkas and Anthony 1989; Liberman 1987). In development of psychosocial programs, families have been enlisted as advocates, paid and unpaid staff, and independent developers of programs. Because there have been disagreements about the role of families in service delivery, as indicated earlier, attitude surveys, impact studies, and research on appropriate training models are needed. At present, it seems that many family groups are willing to assume a valuable adjunctive role to the provider system. It thus becomes important to conceptualize and test new service models involving pooled resources of public and private sectors and perhaps new manpower training roles.

An essential correlate of such developments will involve clinical training models aimed at developing a parity perspective in the relations of professionals and families. Several chapters and their commentaries in this book discuss the contributions of family members to clinical education. To date, most have been administered by persons with professional credentials who have a mentally ill relative. However, in various parts of the country, there are increasing uses of other family members as key informants to detail for students the experiential aspects of living with mental illness. Follow-up assessments of the therapeutic sensitivity and skills of students trained under family exposure versus nonexposure conditions will be of considerable interest.

There are also specialized training programs, such as that developed by Hatfield (1983a), that convey the family experiences together with informed models of specific ways in which professionals may be most beneficial to family members. Hatfield's educational programs for families warrant controlled comparisons with psychoeducational interventions in terms of cost-effectiveness and client satisfaction.

CONCLUDING REMARKS ON CLINICAL TRAINING

Many of the suggestions advanced here involve a substantive revision in our conceptualization of disciplinary boundaries and the parameters of clinical training. In actuality, boundaries have already proved to be highly permeable. The distinctions between "clinical" and "counseling" techniques have become increasingly blurred in actual practice in community mental health programs. The counterposing of terms such as educational, psychoeducational, supportive, psychosocial, and the like may muddy the waters further or, alternatively, demonstrate basic commonalities among previously differentiated therapeutic techniques.

Increasingly evident is the trend toward short-term, supportive psychotherapeutic interventions as opposed to the long-term, personality-reconstruction models of earlier years. This became a pragmatic necessity with the expansion of community mental health services to lower-income, less educated, and ethnically diverse clienteles (Lefley and Bestman 1984). The briefer supportive models proved to be generally as useful as the more time-costly efforts, and in some cases more effective (Gunderson et al. 1984).

We are now approaching a watershed era in psychotherapy, with diminishing federal supports and a turn toward marketing mental health services and developing innovative areas of consumer demand. Stress management models have already begun to supplant insight therapies. Psychoeducational interventions have proved more responsive to the needs of families of chronic patients than have family systems approaches. A substantial number of mental health agencies have begun to approach NAMI affiliates with offers to provide facilities and professional backup for family support groups. There are state-level incentives for local clinics to involve families in planning service models for aftercare of patients. Families have become involved in advisory and governance boards, and even in planning new directions for clinical training.

The research directions suggested in this chapter are oriented toward developing a revised conceptualization of families among new generations of mental health professionals. The general hypothesis is obviously that more rigorous investigations of some old questions, with alternative hypotheses or new explanatory models, will yield a more positive picture of families than the one we still perceive in clinical training and in the professional literature. In particular, it is believed that a focus on strengths and coping skills, rather than on pathogenesis, will yield empirically based models for involving families more effectively in the total therapeutic process.

References

Alanen YO: The family in the pathogenesis of schizophrenic and neurotic disorders. Acta Psychiatr Scand 42 (suppl 189), 1966

Anderson CM, Reiss DJ, Hogarty GE: Schizophrenia and the Family. New York, Guilford, 1986

Angermeyer NC: "Normal deviance"—changing norms under abnormal circumstances, in Psychiatry, The State of the Art, Vol 7. Edited by Pichot P, Berner P, Wolf R, et al. New York, Plenum, 1985, pp 473–479

Anthony EJ: The impact of mental and physical illness on family life. Am J Psychiatry 127:136–143, 1970

Appleton WS: Mistreatment of patients' families by psychiatrists. Am J Psychiatry 131:655–657, 1974

Arey S, Warheit GJ: Psychosocial costs of living with psychologically disturbed family members, in The Social Consequences of Psychiatric Illness. Edited by Robins L, Clayton P, Wing JK. New York, Brunner/Mazel, 1980, pp 158–175

Arnoff FN: Social consequences of policy toward mental illness. Science 188:1277–1281, 1975

Ascher-Svanum H, Sobel TS: Caregivers of mentally ill adults: a woman's agenda. Hosp Community Psychiatry 40:843–845, 1989

Beardslee WR, Podorefsky S: Resilient adolescents whose parents have serious affective and other disorders: importance of self-understanding and relationships. Am J Psychiatry 145:63–68, 1988

Berkowitz R, Kuipers L, Eberlein-Frief R, et al: Lowering expressed emotion in relatives of schizophrenics, in New Developments in Interventions With Families of Schizophrenics (New Directions for Mental Health Services, No 12). Edited by Goldstein MJ. San Francisco, CA, Jossey-Bass, 1981, pp 27–48

Bernal G, Deegan E, Konjevich C: The EPPI family therapy outcome study. International Journal of Family Therapy 5:3–21, 1983

Bernheim KF, Lehman AF: Working With Families of the Mentally Ill. New York, WW Norton, 1985

Blakar RM: Psychopathology and familial communication, in The Structure of Action. Edited by Brenner M. Oxford, Basil Blackwell, 1980

Breier A, Strauss J: Self-control in psychotic disorders. Arch Gen Psychiatry 40:1141–1145, 1983

Breznitz S: Chores as a buffer against risky interaction. Schizophr Bull 11:357–360, 1985

Brown G, Harris TO: Social Origins of Depression: A Study of Psychiatric Disorder in Women. New York, Free Press, 1978

Caplan PJ, Hall-McCorquodale I: Mother-blaming in major clinical journals. Am J Orthopsychiatry 55:345–353, 1985a

Caplan PJ, Hall-McCorquodale I: The scapegoating of mothers: a call for change. Am J Orthopsychiatry 55:610–613, 1985b

Cheek FE: Family interaction patterns and convalescent adjustment of the schizophrenic. Arch Gen Psychiatry 13:138–142, 1965

Chess S: The "blame the mother" ideology. International Journal of Mental Health 11:95–107, 1982

Clausen JA, Yarrow MR: The impact of mental illness on the family. Journal of Social Issues 11:1–65, 1955

Coursey RD: Psychotherapy with persons suffering from schizophrenia: the need for a new agenda. Schizophr Bull 15:349–353, 1989

Culbertson FM: The search for help of parents of autistic children or beware of professional "groupthink." Journal of Clinical Child Psychology 6:63–65, 1977

Dell PF: Researching the family theories of schizophrenia: an exercise in epistemological confusion. Fam Process 19:321–335, 1980

Dohrenwend BP, Dohrenwend BS, Gould MS, et al: Mental Illness in the United States: Epidemiological Estimates. New York, Praeger, 1980

Doll W: Family coping with the mentally ill: an unanticipated problem of deinstitutionalization. Hosp Community Psychiatry 27:183–185, 1976

Falloon IRH, Boyd JL, McGill CW: Family Care of Schizophrenia. New York, Guilford, 1984

Farkas MD, Anthony W (eds): Psychiatric Rehabilitation Programs: Putting Theory Into Practice. Baltimore, MD, Johns Hopkins University Press, 1989

Figley CR, McCubbin HI (eds): Stress and the Family, Vol 2: Coping With Catastrophe. New York, Brunner/Mazel, 1983

Gardos G, Cole JO, LaBrie RA: A 12-year follow-up study of chronic schizophrenics. Hosp Community Psychiatry 33:983–984, 1982

Garmezy N, Rutter M (eds): Stress, Coping, and Development in Children. New York, McGraw-Hill, 1983

Giel R, de Arango NV, Babikir AH, et al: The burden of mental illness on the family: results of observations in four developing countries. Acta Psychiatr Scand 68:186–201, 1983

Group for the Advancement of Psychiatry: A family affair—helping families cope with mental illness: a guide for the professions (Rep No 119). New York, Brunner/Mazel, 1986

Grunebaum H, Weiss JL, Cohler BJ, et al: Mentally Ill Mothers and Their Children, 2nd Edition. Chicago, IL, University of Chicago Press, 1982

Gunderson JG, Frank AF, Katz HM, et al: Effects of psychotherapy in schizophrenia, II: comparative outcome of two forms of treatment. Schizophr Bull 10:564–598, 1984

Haley J: Leaving Home. New York, McGraw-Hill, 1980

Hatfield AB: Psychological costs of schizophrenia to the family. Social Work 23:355–359, 1978

Hatfield AB: Coping With Mental Illness in the Family: A Family Guide. Arlington, VA, National Alliance for the Mentally Ill, 1983a

Hatfield AB: What families want of family therapists, in Family Therapy in Schizophrenia. Edited by McFarlane WR. New York, Guilford, 1983b, pp 41–65

Hatfield AB, Lefley HP: Families of the Mentally Ill: Coping and Adaptation. New York, Guilford, 1987

Hatfield AB, Spaniol L, Zipple AM: Expressed emotion: a family perspective. Schizophr Bull 13:221–226, 1987

Herz MI: Recognizing and preventing relapse in patients with schizophrenia. Hosp Community Psychiatry 35:344–349, 1984

Herz MI, Endicott J, Spitzer RL: Brief versus standard hospitalization: the families. Am J Psychiatry 133:795–801, 1976

Hirsch SR: Do parents cause schizophrenia? Trends in Neurosciences 2:49–52, 1979

Hirsch SR, Leff JP: Abnormalities in Parents of Schizophrenics. London, Oxford University Press, 1975

Hoffman L: Foundations of Family Therapy. New York, Basic Books, 1981

Holden DF, Lewine RRJ: How families evaluate mental health professionals, resources, and effects of illness. Schizophr Bull 8:626–633, 1982

Holmes TH, Rahe RH: The social readjustment rating scale. J Psychosom Res 11:213–218, 1967

Howe JW: What do families of citizens with mental illness want from clinicians? Tie-Lines 2:8–9, 1985

Howells JG, Guirguis WR: The Family and Schizophrenia. New York, International Universities Press, 1985

Jenkins JH, Karno M, de la Selva A, et al: Expressed emotion in cross-cultural context: familial responses to schizophrenia among Mexican Americans, in Treatment of Schizophrenia: Family Assessment and Intervention. Edited by Goldstein MJ. Berlin, Springer-Verlag, 1986, pp 35–49

Kanter JS: Consulting with families of the chronic mentally ill, in Clinical Issues in Treating the Chronic Mentally Ill (New Directions for Mental Health Services, No 27). Edited by Kanter JS. San Francisco, CA, Jossey-Bass, 1985a, pp 21–32

Kanter JS: Moral issues and mental illness, in Clinical Issues in Treating the Chronic Mentally Ill (New Directions for Mental Health Services, No 27). Edited by Kanter JS. San Francisco, CA, Jossey-Bass, 1985b, pp 47–62

Kanter JS: The process of change in the long-term mentally ill: a naturalistic perspective. Psychosocial Rehabilitation Journal 9:55–69, 1985c

Kauffman C, Grunebaum H, Vohler B, et al: Superkids: competent children of psychotic mothers. Am J Psychiatry 136:1398–1402, 1979

Keller MB, Beardslee WR, Dorer DJ, et al: Impact of severity and chronicity of parental affective illness on adaptive functioning and psychopathology of children. Arch Gen Psychiatry 43:930–937, 1986

Kessler RC, Price RH, Wortman CB: Social factors in psychopathology: stress, social support, and coping processes. Ann Rev Psychol 36:531–572, 1985

Kety SS: Comments on the NIMH-Israeli high-risk study. Schizophr Bull 11:354–356, 1985

Klerman GL: Ideology and science in the individual psychotherapy of schizophrenia. Schizophr Bull 10:608–612, 1984

Kreisman DE, Joy VD: Family response to the mental illness of a relative: a review of the literature. Schizophr Bull 1:34–54, 1974

Lamb HR: Families: practical help replaces blame. Hosp Community Psychiatry 34:893, 1983

Leff J: Psychiatry Around the Globe: A Transcultural View. New York, Marcel Dekker, 1981

Lefley HP: Delivering mental health services across cultures, in Mental Health Services: The Cultural Context. Edited by Pedersen PB, Sartorius N, Marsella AM. New York, Sage, 1984, pp 135–171

Lefley HP: Etiological and prevention views of clinicians with mentally ill relatives. Am J Orthopsychiatry 55:363–370, 1985a

Lefley HP: Families of the mentally ill in cross-cultural perspective. Psychosocial Rehabilitation Journal 8:57–75, 1985b

Lefley HP: Why cross-cultural training? Applied issues in culture and mental health service delivery, in Cross-Cultural Training for Mental Health Professionals. Edited by Lefley HP, Pedersen PB. Springfield, IL, Charles C Thomas, 1986, pp 11–44

Lefley HP: Aging parents as caregivers of mentally ill adult children: an emerging social problem. Hosp Community Psychiatry 38:1063–1070, 1987a

Lefley HP: Culture and mental illness: the family role, in Families of the Mentally Ill: Coping and Adaptation. Edited by Hatfield AB, Lefley HP. New York, Guilford, 1987b, pp 30–59

Lefley HP: Impact of mental illness in families of mental health professionals. J Nerv Ment Dis 175:613–619, 1987c

Lefley HP, Bestman EW: Community mental health and minorities: a multiethnic approach, in The Pluralistic Society: A Community Mental Health Perspective. Edited by Sue S, Moore T. New York, Human Sciences Press, 1984, pp 116–148

Liberman RP: Psychiatric Rehabilitation of Chronic Mental Patients. Washington, DC, American Psychiatric Press, 1987

Liem JH: Family studies of schizophrenia: an update and commentary. Schizophr Bull 6:429–455, 1980

McCubbin HI, Figley CR (eds): Stress and the Family, Vol 1: Coping With Normative Transitions. New York, Brunner/Mazel, 1983

McFarlane WR: Multiple family therapy in schizophrenia, in Family Therapy in Schizophrenia. Edited by McFarlane WR, Beels CC. New York, Guilford, 1983, pp 141–172

McFarlane WR, Beels CC: Family research in schizophrenia: a review and integration for clinicians, in Family Therapy in Schizophrenia. Edited by McFarlane WR, Beels CC. New York, Guilford, 1983, pp 311–323

McGlashan TH: The Chestnut Lodge follow-up study, II: long-term outcome of schizophrenia and the affective disorders. Arch Gen Psychiatry 41:586–601, 1984

Maranhao T: Family therapy and anthropology. Cult Med Psychiatry 8:255–279, 1984

Margolin G: Ethical and legal considerations in marital and family therapy. Am Psychol 37:788–800, 1982

Mirsky AF, Silberman EK, Latz A, et al: Adult outcome of high-risk children: differential effects of town and kibbutz rearing. Schizophr Bull 11:150–154, 1985

Moline RA, Singh S, Morris A, et al: Family expressed emotion and relapse in schizophrenia in 24 urban American patients. Am J Psychiatry 142:1078–1081, 1985

Mosher LR, Keith SJ: Psychosocial treatment: individual, groups, family, and community support approaches, in Special Report: Schizophrenia, 1980. Washington, DC, U.S. Government Printing Office, 1981

Noh S, Turner RJ: Living with psychiatric patients: implications for the mental health of family members. Soc Sci Med 25:263–271, 1987

Parker G: Re-searching the schizophrenogenic mother. J Nerv Ment Dis 170:452–462, 1982

Pearlin LI, Lieberman MA, Meneghan EG, et al: The stress process. J Health Soc Behav 22:337–356, 1981

Platt S: Measuring the burden of psychiatric illness on the family: an evaluation of some rating scales. Psychol Med 15:383–393, 1985

Reiss D: The family and schizophrenia. Am J Psychiatry 133:181–185, 1976

Reynolds D, Farberow NL: The Family Shadow: Sources of Suicide and Schizophrenia. Berkeley, University of California Press, 1981

Rice EP, Ekdahl MC, Miller L: Children of Mentally Ill Parents. New York, Behavioral Publications, 1971

Ruocchio PJ: How psychotherapy can help the schizophrenic patient. Hosp Community Psychiatry 40:188–190, 1989

Samuels L, Chase L: The well siblings of schizophrenics. American Journal of Family Therapy 7:24–35, 1979

Schuman M: The Bowen theory and the hospitalized patient, in Family Interventions With Psychiatric Patients. Edited by Luber RF, Anderson CM. New York, Human Sciences Press, 1983, pp 29–47

Shaver KG: The Attribution of Blame. New York, Springer-Verlag, New York, 1985

Spaniol L, Jung H, Zipple A, et al: Families as a central resource in the rehabilitation of the severely psychiatrically disabled: report of a national survey. Boston University, Center for Rehabilitation Research & Training in Mental Health, Boston, MA, 1984

Stone MH: Etiological factors in schizophrenia: a reevaluation in the light of contemporary research. Psychiatr Q 50:83–119, 1978

Terkelsen KG: Schizophrenia and the family, II: adverse effects of family therapy. Fam Process 22:191–200, 1983

Terkelsen KG, Cole SA: Methodological flaws in the schizophrenogenic hypothesis and their implications for mental health services in an era of community care. Unpublished paper, Family Institute of Westchester, Mount Vernon, NY, 1985

Thoits PA: Dimensions of life events that influence psychological distress: an evaluation and synthesis of the literature, in Psychosocial Stress: Trends in Theory and Research. Edited by Kaplan HB. New York, Academic, 1983

Thompson EH, Doll W: The burden of families coping with the mentally ill: an invisible crisis. Family Relations 31:379–388, 1982

Thurer SL: Deinstitutionalization and women: where the buck stops. Hosp Community Psychiatry 34:1162–1163, 1983

Torrey EF: Surviving Schizophrenia: A Family Manual, Revised Edition. New York, Harper & Row, 1988

Turnbull AP, Turnbull HR: Parents Speak Out: Views From the Other Side of the Two-Way Mirror. Columbus, OH, Charles E Merrill, 1978

Vaughn CE, Snyder KS, Jones S, et al: Family factors in schizophrenic relapse. Arch Gen Psychiatry 41:1169–1177, 1984

Wasow M: Chronic schizophrenia and Alzheimer's disease: the losses for parents, spouses, and children compared. J Chronic Dis 38:711–716, 1985

Wechsler JA, Schwartztol HW, Wechsler NF: In a Darkness: A Story of Young Suicide, 2nd Edition. Miami, FL, Pickering Press, 1988

Wig NN, Menon K, Bedi H, et al: Distribution of expressed emotion components among relatives of schizophrenic patients in Aarhus and Chandigarh. Br J Psychiatry 151:160–165, 1987

World Health Organization: The International Pilot Study of Schizophrenia, Vol 1. Geneva, Switzerland, WHO, 1973

World Health Organization: Schizophrenia: An International Follow-Up Study. Chichester, England, John Wiley, 1979

Commentary to Chapter 5

How Goes the Battle?

Samuel J. Keith, M.D.
H. Alice Lowery, Ph.D.

We have frequently heard that schizophrenia will alter the expectations of 3 million Americans during the course of their lifetimes—3 million Americans who will experience the onset of an illness that will decrease and far too often eliminate the possibility of completing an education, beginning a career, or enjoying a life once filled with promise. Many will continue an existence without control of that most human of qualities—the human mind, with its unique ability to distinguish reality from fantasy, friend from foe, joy from sadness. Yet, as Dr. Lefley has pointed out to us in her eloquent chapter, the 3 million Americans bearing the diagnosis are far from being the only people who have suffered the scourge of schizophrenia. Each person suffering from schizophrenia has two parents and, on average, at least one sibling, raising the total at a minimum to 12 million Americans who are schizophrenic or who have suffered from the effects of schizophrenia. If we add spouses, children, other close relatives, and friends, the suffering caused by schizophrenia increases exponentially. Along with the illness and the personal and familial suffering and disability that it causes comes an enormous cost to our society; a cost as significant as atherosclerotic heart disease or cancer; a cost compounded by ignorance and fear.

Much of this fear and ignorance about schizophrenia was driven by etiologic theories that, as identified by Dr. Lefley, focused on the familial etiology as generating, precipitating, or exacerbating the illness. Much of Dr. Lefley's chapter is dedicated to a thorough and systematic examination of what was wrong with the early research in terms of its tautological hypotheses, which ignored such issues as direction of effect, inappropriateness of measurement, and variability

163

of outcome. Dr. Lefley then proposed what kind of research would correct for the mistakes of the past. I agree with Dr. Lefley's evaluation and add some additional thoughts. For example, in the assessment of stressful life events, she is correct in saying that chronic stress is rarely considered. Further, most measurements of stress consider those stresses that occur; they fail to take into account those stresses that result from things that were expected to happen, but that did not; for example, the loss of a life once filled with promise. Coping with psychotic symptoms and all the related stress (and this is not meant to minimize it) generally requires action that may be easier to some extent than the demoralizing effects of the negative symptoms—the withdrawal and loss of will, goal-directed behavior, and affect—which grind excruciatingly onward, seemingly unresponsive to any approach.

The study of chronic stress in families of the chronically mentally ill necessitates the development of better instruments for its assessment. In fact, the study of coping strengths will also require new instrumentation. The existence of events does not necessarily mean a concurrent and equal experience of stress related to the event. The availability and use of coping mechanisms provides a potentially powerful modifier variable against experiencing stress.

We could spend the rest of our time discussing Dr. Lefley's chapter, agreeing with what she said, and adding bits and pieces, but we would like to attempt something a little different. It is our sense that Dr. Lefley does not take her chapter far enough in stating the potential of the role of research on the family. The iatrogenic damage to patients and their families is the result of a misinformed era of understanding about schizophrenia. Unfortunately, the historical antecedents of assignment of blame in the absence of data are many. Moral infirmities, demonic possession, and schizophrenogenic mothers are all examples of this phenomenon. And, yes, we have all seen the results of contemporary de Torquemadas. The anguish caused by people who were wrong is no less painful because they believed they were doing the right thing. Dr. Lefley calls for research to demonstrate the adverse effects on families—Do the ways a therapist reacts in causing anger and humiliation have a negative impact on families and does this impact in turn have a negative impact on the patient? Of course it does. Dr. Lefley and others in this book cite anecdote after anecdote of damaging, unethical, immoral actions made under the rubrics of treatment. The question remains, however, Will systematic study of this damage result in a change in clinical treatment? Anecdotes are dangerous—it is just this kind of evidence that led to so much damage being perpetrated on families; it is this kind of evidence that led to the polarization of families and professionals; it is this kind of evidence that perpetuates the mistakes of the past, by extending them into the future. We need not emulate a practice whose failures we condemn. There has never been an excuse for harmful, unethical, immoral behavior in the form of psychiatric treatment. It needs not to be studied; it needs to be stopped.

It is here that our major questions for Dr. Lefley occur. Would it be better to try to undo the damage of the generation of familial etiology for schizophrenia, or would we be better advised to direct our major effort at educating clinicians on the current data about schizophrenia? Perhaps this is a defensive response to the damage that has already been done. Perhaps George Santayana's position— those who forget history are condemned to repeat it—is correct. But can a more positive approach be taken as well? If we are able to provide an education that supports the position that schizophrenia is an illness with a genetic component as strong as any other medical illness, we move toward a position of dignity and respect for those who have so long labored with insufficient tools to help their family members and who bear the double punishment of an illness and an accusation of causality. It is not that in taking this position we have obviated the need to look at environmental issues in the course of illness. Nor does it need to encourage the forgetting of history. There are certain to be environmental factors that are helpful and those that are not. Dr. Lefley's own career interest in the impact of cross-cultural differences would argue that, of course, the environment is important in outcome. This is true of such illnesses as epilepsy, stroke, hypertension, and diabetes—we should expect it to be true of schizophrenia. What is different in teaching about schizophrenia as an illness is that an atheoretical, data-oriented approach can be taken that avoids premature and inappropriate closure on causality.

For example, in our treatment of schizophrenia, which we acknowledge is not adequate, Dr. Lefley criticizes the current state of knowledge about conflicting literatures on even the role of medication and the confusion this creates in families. Unfortunately, this problem is not confined to schizophrenia but is clear in such treatments as steroids for arthritis, coronary bypass surgery for compromised arteries, and many of the treatments for cancer. The solution, however, is to hold clinicians responsible for providing a clear presentation of data—not myth, not belief system, not what they read 15 years ago— to families and patients so that informed decisions can be made by a clinical treatment team that includes the clinician, the patient, and the family. In our treatment approach, we also must be aware that schizophrenia is not a homogeneous illness by diagnosis nor is there a homogeneous treatment that will always be helpful. Schizophrenia is an illness most likely of striking heterogeneity of causality. Further, the course of the illness as experienced by a group or by an individual is clearly variable. As a patient passes through various phases—acute psychosis, early stabilization, recovery—he or she will have differing needs from treatment and from the environment. In fact, we are dealing with an illness of such monumental variability that it is remarkable that group differences appear at all. That they do, for example, in the role of neuroleptics, the role of psychoeducation, and the role of skills training for families and patients argues for our current path being correct but needing refinement.

Some investigators have tried to make the point that they are concerned with environmental factors, found in the therapeutic environment as well as the natural environment, that have been implicated in the relapse of some schizophrenic patients. Hogarty et al. (1986) postulated that "there was a *commonality* among the offending stimuli that were contained in the natural and the therapeutic environments of patients—a commonality that required the vulnerable patient to make an adaptive response to complex, vague, multiple, or emotionally charged expectations" (p. 634). One factor that has received considerable attention is expressed emotion (EE).

The apparent robustness of the EE findings raises a number of questions, one of which is whether there is a genetic component to the EE phenomenon. Ming Tsuang suggested that future research should distinguish the psychosocial, biological, and genetic components of the phenomenon. For example, neuropsychological measures such as eye tracking could be used to quantify and characterize high and low EE in an effort to tease apart components. Work in this area is being carried out by Diane Wagner and her colleagues at Pittsburgh. Preliminary evidence reported by Hogarty et al. (1986) suggests that information-processing deficits are more likely to appear among siblings in high-EE households than among siblings in low-EE households.

As Dr. Lefley has indicated, we need to learn more about high and low EE. In addition to questions she raised (e.g., what are the personality correlates and antecedents of EE), we need to know the parameters of the constructs: Is there variability in the level of EE cross-culturally? Data from Jenkins et al. (1986) suggest that there might be. However, the lower level of EE found in her Mexican American sample could have been due to the larger number of females in this sample than in Vaughn et al.'s (1984) Anglo-Saxon sample. Hogarty et al. (1986) have suggested that the major EE results may be specific to males. Moline et al. (1985) suggested lower levels of EE among blacks; however, the investigators themselves raised numerous questions about the quality of their data. Other questions include: How is EE influenced by changes in the patient's behavior?

What is the direction of the effect? How stable is the measure of EE? How do different components of EE interact with clinical state? What are the positive and negative components of EE? What is the rate of critical-intrusive environments outside the family? John Wing (personal communication) reported that iatrogenic EE is what he may have captured in his study of "total push" rehabilitation in which he was able to bring about striking relapse rates in formerly remitted patients (Wing et al. 1972).

It is clear from the accumulation of data from the EE studies that whatever the initial impetus was for the EE work, it has become an important area for study in our attempt to understand environmental—not necessarily familial—elements in recovery. The family environment as an in vivo laboratory should not become exclusive or totally inclusive in the implication of the findings. EE, for example, is not unique to families, it is alterable through education, and in some preliminary reports it may have a differential impact depending on the phase of the illness or the type of outcome being assessed. It has been suggested that high EE may indeed be associated with relapse, but that relapse, per se, is not the only measure of outcome we should be considering. The "benign indifference" argued for by Anderson et al. (1986) may be the best approach during a recovery from acute psychosis, but is it best for recovery from the negative-symptom state seen later in the course of illness? Will low EE at that point in the recovery period be encouraging of a continuation of a pattern of the deficit state of schizophrenia?

Looking at the whole issue of continuity of care and stages of treatment from the acute phase through recovery might be highly advantageous. It would allow us to identify major gaps in our knowledge regarding treatment and rehabilitation of schizophrenic patients as well as the more promising areas needing further development. Of relevance to this issue is Stein and Test's (1985) conclusion in developing and evaluating their training in community living model: the strategies of cure in preparing people for life after treatment are not effective for patients suffering from chronic or lifelong illness. In their view, the more appropriate strategy accepts the reality that we do not know how to prevent or cure chronic mental illness, but that techniques exist that allow the disorder to be managed well. Integration of families into the entire process, in all stages of treatment, from active to supportive roles, would be mutually advantageous.

The importance of extending our knowledge about the environment in recovery from schizophrenia is relevant not just to schizophrenia but as a model for other illnesses. As a model of an illness, will it not be possible to transfer the knowledge we gain from its study to other illnesses to make the recovery easier or even the defeat by disease less painful?

Central in our discussion is that schizophrenia can be discussed from an illness model, and educating clinicians about it from this perspective will permit an entirely different perspective on the role of families. It will eliminate the destructive blaming of families that has accompanied no other illness as it has schizophrenia. But it will not be enough to teach about it from this perspective any more than the examination of a cancer cell under a microscope provides an understanding of the illness of cancer. Clinicians need to experience the impact of chronic illness. Current undergraduate medical training where critical opinions develop about illnesses, for example, provides only cross-sectional slices through chronic illness by virtue of time-limited clerkships or hospital-based exposure. What this accomplishes is exposure to the acute presentations of all illnesses, e.g., diabetes, arthritis, cancer, and schizophrenia. And yet, the acute presentation, as Dr. Lefley has stated so well, is not the source of the majority of pain for either patients or families. How much better it would be for a young medical student's education and empathy to be given a longitudinal assignment to follow a patient with a chronic illness, regardless of the type, throughout his or her training career. How much more a student would learn over a 4-year period by going to the patient's family home to see how chronic illness truly affects the lives of people. A discharge from a hospital or a rotation onto a new clerkship should not limit a student's understanding about the impact of illness.

The process Dr. Lefley has initiated is correct in redressing the wrongs of the past. We are in a position to redress these mistakes by combining a positive position on how the next decade of research and education will contribute to better lives for all afflicted by mental illness with an understanding of the mistakes of the past. It is time to put aside the battles of the past that have unfortunately left so many scars on so many people. In another place, in another time, the process and outcome of this type of battle were addressed quite eloquently by Horatio, whose commander sent a messenger to ask, "How goes the battle, Horatio?"

"Tell him," Horatio responded, "the battle goes well, it is the troops who truly suffer."

REFERENCES

Anderson CM, Reiss DJ, Hogarty GE: Schizophrenia and the Family. New York, Guilford, 1986

Hogarty GE, Anderson CM, Reiss DJ, et al: Family psychoeducation, social skills training, and maintenance chemotherapy in the aftercare treatment of schizophrenia. Arch Gen Psychiatry 43:633–642, 1986

Jenkins JH, Karno M, de la Selva A, et al: Expressed emotion in cross-cultural context: familial responses to schizophrenia among Mexican-Americans, in Treatment of Schizophrenia: Family Assessment and Intervention. Edited by Goldstein MJ. Berlin, Springer-Verlag, 1986, pp 35–49

Moline RA, Singh S, Morris A, et al: Family expressed emotion and relapse in schizophrenia in 24 urban American patients. Am J Psychiatry 142:1078–1081, 1985

Stein LI, Test MA (eds): The Training in Community Living Model: a Decade of Experience (New Directions for Mental Health Services, No 26). San Francisco, CA, Jossey-Bass, 1985

Vaughn CE, Snyder KS, Jones S, et al: Family factors in schizophrenic relapse. Arch Gen Psychiatry 41:1169–1177, 1984

Wing L, Wing JK, Griffiths D, et al: An epidemiological and experimental evaluation of industrial rehabilitation of chronic psychotic patients in the community, in Evaluating a Community Psychiatric Service. Edited by Wing JK, Hailey AM. London, Oxford University Press, 1972, pp 359–404

Part II

Models for Educating Professionals

Ethical and Legal Considerations for Interviewing Families of the Seriously Mentally Ill

Evelyn McElroy, R.N., Ph.D.

Distress for families who have relatives with a major mental illness such as the schizophrenias or the major affective disorders evolves from four possible sources. The first source of distress involves learning that someone valued has a serious illness and that the prognosis is questionable. A second source of distress for families evolves from alterations in goals and life changes that the relative's illness has created when thorough diagnostic evaluations and observations have established that the illness may be chronic. A third source of distress occurs if resources to meet the altered life plans are insufficient. A fourth potential source of distress among families is created by some mental health professionals as a result of practices that disregard the ethical and human rights of families to dignity, privacy, and informed consent regarding treatments involving them.

This chapter addresses transactions and interviewing practices used by some professionals that have caused extreme, unnecessary distress and have increased the burden of many families in crisis.

Special thanks are given to Henry Harbin, M.D., for reading an earlier version of this chapter and to Diana Katachadourian of the Classics Department of Johns Hopkins University for helping to research the Greek derivatives of the hygosystogenic concept.

Names have been changed and other slight changes have been made to the cases presented in this chapter to provide anonymity for the Doe and the Jones families.

Guidelines are proposed for mental health professionals to use when interviewing families of the seriously mentally ill. Recommendations are made for families and professionals to consider when unethical or potentially illegal interviewing practices by other staff members compromise the dignity, privacy, or human rights of individuals with relatives in psychiatric settings. Curriculum content to augment the educational preparation of mental health professionals is recommended. Recommendations are proposed to study issues of concern to families who must interact with representatives of the mental health care delivery system. Finally, changes are proposed for some systems that provide service or evaluate psychiatric hospitals or facilities.

CASE EXAMPLES

The Doe Incident

Why is it necessary to devote attention to the ways in which families are interviewed by professionals in mental health settings? A letter from the mother of a 17-year-old patient illustrates the importance of addressing the topic and proposing guidelines for interviewing families as an initial step in preventing unnecessary distress and developing effective ways of establishing a therapeutic alliance between professionals and families. The purpose of such an alliance is to support the treatment and rehabilitation plan of the patient.

The adolescent described in the following letter had functioned well in school, was popular, and was active in extracurricular activities before the sudden onset of psychotic symptoms. Thorough diagnostic testing, consultations, and treatment in private hospitals for 80% of the next 2 years resulted in little improvement, and chronic schizophrenia was diagnosed. This letter was written 18 months after the onset of the illness.

Dr. X
Director, Psychiatry
Private Psychiatric Hospital
Anytown, USA

Dear Dr. X:

Last Wednesday at approximately 3:10 I met with staff member A and family therapy consultant B for the purpose of determining their perspective on treating families and to explore issues of confidentiality should my husband and I decide to participate in that treatment modality as one aspect of the treatment rendered to my son, John, who is an inpatient at your facility. During the course of our interview, I revealed some information which was sensitive to me which pertained to the objectives of our meeting. Approximately 10 minutes later I was informed that other persons were viewing the session in a manner that resulted in an unauthorized invasion of my privacy and violated the confidentiality and trust that is inherent in any kind of therapeutic contract between professionals and clients.

You should know that my husband and I have been impressed with many of the other members of your staff. We have been particularly touched by the sensitive and professional way in which staff member J has related to both our son and ourselves. Dr. C has consistently responded to our needs in a timely, warm, and helpful manner. The evening staff has always made us feel welcome as we visited John and we are indebted to Dr. D for helping us obtain help at the hospital when we needed it. I mention this because you should know when your staff is performing effectively and well. That is why it is particularly distressing to cope with the incident today. It is a travesty to have an effective therapeutic relationship unnecessarily compromised by irresponsible behavior on the part of some persons.

I do not like to have my feelings and concerns treated in such a cavalier fashion by insensitive people. I will not be treated in such an undignified manner nor will I allow my human and legal rights to be so flagrantly violated. I am interested in obtaining the names of the persons present at the session, their relationship to the inpatient unit, and their discipline.

I am interested in learning from you about suggestions to ensure that other families in crisis are not further traumatized by those charged with helping them.

Sincerely,

Jane Doe

The family therapy consultant involved was an experienced family systems expert who was on the faculty of a university with responsibility for introducing mental health professionals to the technique of family systems approaches. In the incident described, she was teaching four other professionals. She was the role model.

It is of interest that none of the "eavesdroppers" who were observing the transactions interrupted the session. All were aware that Mrs. Doe's privacy had been violated and that informed consent had not been obtained. The four professionals consisted of two mental health workers, a master's-prepared psychiatric nurse, and a psychiatrist. One of the mental health workers and the family therapy consultant had agreed to meet with the parent.

One can only ponder at the implementation of such unethical professional practices from the family systems therapist and the mental health worker and at the failure of those observing to respond in ways commensurate with the ethical codes of practice inherent in their respective disciplines. The family therapy consultant was concerned with engaging the parent in family therapy because the son had experienced frequent relapses. The family therapy consultant felt the family's high level of emotional expression (EE) contributed to the relapses. This assumption was later revealed to be incorrect as the youngster had been misdiagnosed. When prescribed lithium and carbamazepine to control his rapid cyclic disorder, he was able to progress successfully in age-appropriate tasks without further relapses. The long-lasting effect of the medication to control the symptoms of the disease along with continued residence with the family through college suggests that factors other than their interpersonal style contributed to the symptoms. Informed consent is the most important issue at question in the incident.

Informed consent on practices affecting families.   The goal of informed consent is the protection of the rights of individuals subjected to treatment (Breggin 1979). According to Plotkin (1977),

> Informed consent exists when the following three conditions are met: the physician makes a reasonable disclosure to the patient of treatment risks; a voluntary decision is made by the patient based on this disclosure; and the patient is competent to make such a decision. These three elements—disclosure, voluntariness, and competency— clearly apply to a psychiatrist's use of previously discussed [psychosurgery, psychotropic drugs, and behavior therapy].

In the Doe incident, the parent was never given full disclosure of the therapy, was not given a choice about whether she wanted to be observed by others, was never informed of the risks, and was denied her right to make a voluntary decision. The potential hazards of such treatment included the development of adverse psychological symptoms that persisted and contributed to distress and directly increased the burden faced by the mother. Furthermore, such behaviors could jeopardize the therapeutic alliance among other staff working with the patient, which could result in possible withdrawal of the patient from treatment.

The Doe incident was rated as a 5, the highest score possible, on a Likert-type scale designed to measure situational distress created by the interview. Three years after the incident, the parent continued to feel enraged and distraught by the event. During the interim, she sought treatment for a stress-related disorder, and she perceived the interview to be a contributing event to her disorder. The interview should be viewed as having caused significant psychological trauma.

Ethical and legal implications.   The confidentiality of a privileged relationship as described in Section 8 of the *Principles of Medical Ethics of the American Medical Association* (1954) was violated. The confidentiality of the doctor-patient relationship is recognized by both the medical and legal professions. The actions violated the Hippocratic oath. Similarly, the incident violated assumptions held by most theories of psychotherapy that agree to the protection of privacy of the interpersonal relationship between the patient and the doctor (or therapist) (Slovenko and Udin 1966; Ruben and Ruben 1972). The situation violated the essence of psychiatric treatment and failed in the preservation of human dignity for the family.

The legal aspects of the incident must be viewed from the perspective of the state in question. The Maryland courts have held that a tort suit may be brought to redress an unwarranted invasion of privacy. In *Beane v. McMullen* (1972), reasonableness under the facts presented was the determining factor in resolution of a lawsuit for invasion of privacy. The requisite elements of tort as defined by the Court of Appeals in *Hollander v. Lubow* were that an invasion of privacy is subject to liability if it is unreasonable and if it would be highly offensive to a reasonable person. Privacy is invaded when there is intrusion on the seclusion of another. In addition, one is subjected to liability when unreasonable invasion of privacy occurs that would be highly offensive to a reasonable person and not of legitimate concern to the public (*Hollander v. Lubow* 1975; Reinstatement Second, Torts, 1975).

According to Prosser and Keeton (1985), the tort of intrusion on one's seclusion has been applied to eavesdropping by means of wire taps and microphones and to looking in the windows of a home. Both varieties of invasion of privacy would appear to be present in the situation described by Mrs. Doe. Furthermore, the unauthorized intrusion on privacy by the three staff members who were observing the session could be viewed as contemporaneous eavesdropping, because allowing students to observe is not a normal or reasonable action performed as an aspect of medical or allied support services for or on behalf of the patient. Contemporaneous eavesdropping of the type described in the situation would appear to be in violation of the Annotated Code of Maryland (HG §§ 4-301–303).

In addition, the court in *Shaw v. Glickman* (1980) upheld the privilege of the psychiatrist to maintain confidential information between himself or herself and the patient. In this perspective, it seems likely that the Maryland courts would find the invasion of privacy occasioned by contemporaneous eavesdropping at a psychiatric interview to be unreasonable and thus tortious. Also, because the therapist made a definite representation to the parent that the interview would occur only between himself and the consulting expert in family therapy, his behavior could be viewed as making a willful misrepresentation in treatment, which is grounds for reprimand, suspension, or revocation of his license to practice under the Annotated Code of Maryland (HO § 14–504). This case was not only unethical but litigious and indicated an insensitive disregard for the dignity of the parent and the violation of her constitutional and legal rights.

The incident did not result in withdrawal of the son from the hospital because another psychiatrist and many of the other staff were helpful to the son. In fact, the helpful psychiatrist was responsible for arriving at a valid diagnosis for the son and prescribing appropriate medication to control his symptoms, thus making progress possible. In addition, this psychiatrist and many of the other staff had effectively worked with the patient and obviously cared for him. The psychiatrist had functioned as an advocate for the patient during a ward meeting when other patients were discounting him. Later, the patient indicated that this behavior on the part of the psychiatrist had great meaning to him. In summary, these were the reasons that the son was not transferred to another hospital as a result of the invasion of the mother's privacy. Nevertheless, the parents felt that they did not have to accept such unethical practices from the professionals at the psychiatric hospital.

Resolution of the situation.   Mrs. Doe sent the letter of objection to the chairman of the Department of Psychiatry and mailed a carbon copy to the chairman of the board of the private, nonprofit hospital. She requested to meet with the chairman of the Department of Psychiatry to explore further why such negative practices occurred. At that time, she informed him that she was sending the letter to a lawyer who had an interest in ethics as related to the socialization of professionals. The lawyer was active in the Hastings Institute and was a prominent legal educator.

At the meeting with the chairman of the Department of Psychiatry, Mrs. Doe requested that the ethical implications of the staff's violations of her rights be addressed at staff in-service meetings and that an attorney provide the professionals with information on the legal implications of their practices in such cases.

The parent indicated that later she would like to speak at an in-service program about the feelings she experienced as a result of the event. Mrs. Doe felt that understanding the family perspective on such matters might result in behavioral change among professionals. The feelings that she experienced were described as distress, loss of self-esteem, and a sense of powerlessness. She also indicated that she felt a great deal of rage toward the professionals involved in violating her rights. She stated that in retrospect the incident seemed like a "psychological gang rape" (Mrs. Doe, personal communication, June 1982). One can assume that such behaviors from professionals did not contribute to a sense of trust.

The Jones Incident

Another example of an interview of a family by mental health professionals illustrates the development of distress and the need to change how some professionals interact with families.

> A mother brought the following grievance to a local NAMI [National Alliance for the Mentally Ill] chapter. Her 19-year-old daughter had been committed to a public hospital for treatment of manic depression and had been involved in legal difficulties as a result of her illness. The psychiatrist who had been directing the family therapy sessions requested a consultation with a family systems therapist located in an area approximately 30 miles from the hospital. The family (both parents and the daughter) agreed to attend the session. The parents picked the daughter up from the hospital and drove to the session one Saturday afternoon.
>
> The psychiatrist, the family therapy consultant, and the three members of the Jones family met at the interviewing room. The family was informed (not asked) by the professionals that the session was being videotaped and that 11 other professionals would be observing. They had not been given the information until after they arrived at the session.
>
> The mother was irate that she had not been informed of the procedures in advance and refused to participate and withdrew from the room. The father and daughter agreed to continue with the session. The session centered on the placement of the daughter after discharge from the hospital. The mother had previously indicated that she wanted the daughter to return home and the daughter also wished to return to the family. The father agreed with the psychiatrist that the daughter should reside elsewhere. When it became evident that a recommendation on the postdischarge placement was being sought by the psychiatrist from the family therapy consultant and the result had important implications for the daughter's future, the mother returned to the session. She later claimed that her decision to join the group was to defend herself and her position (A. Jones, personal communication, April 1983).

Ethical and legal aspects of the Jones incident. A great deal of effort had been expended by the family therapist and the psychiatrist to arrange the interview, as evidenced by the television recording equipment, the notice given to the 11 student observers, and arranging for the family to attend the interview in another city. Yet, written or verbal informed consent obtained from the family in a timely manner was lacking. Neither the parents nor the patient were informed that the session was a consultation to corroborate the psychiatrist's aftercare plan.

The family was not informed in advance that the session was to be videotaped nor was permission obtained for the 11 strangers to view this highly personal and sensitive session. The credentials of the observers were not revealed to the parents in a timely manner nor in a way to allow them to carefully consider if they wanted their family concerns revealed to them. Time is required to assimilate and seriously consider the ramifications of such a procedure. Furthermore, the parents were not asked if they wished to be used to train others.

The family therapist involved had a distinguished reputation and was responsible for training mental health professionals to work with families. The psychiatrist who arranged the interview and who was responsible for the incident was also charged with educating professionals to work with families. Both were professional role models.

The mother rated the session as a 5 on a situational distress scale. This score indicates extreme distress. The mother's eventual willingness to enter the session was later interpreted as sanctioning the event. Mrs. Jones, however, said she only participated to defend her position and to ensure that her perspective was represented in a matter that would have a significant impact on her daughter's future. In other words, her subsequent involvement represented a reluctant engagement under duress. The points discussed previously about the ethical aspects of staff-family interactions apply to this case.

The ethics of professionals placing parents in such undignified and potentially powerless positions in front of their offspring pose questions that are different from the first incident cited. Margolin (1982), Hare-Mustin (1980), and Hare-Mustin et al. (1979) have described some of the moral dilemmas faced by families when one member agrees to family interviews whereas another member objects. The difficulty in managing those "resistant" family members has been addressed (Anderson and Stewart 1983; Walsh 1985). Consideration for resolving dissonance between family and staff regarding family interviews has rarely been directed toward an examination of professionals' behavior to determine if their biases toward families contribute to practices and result in the families rejecting the treatment offered. In addition, the goals of assistance from all family members must be assessed to determine if they are congruent with the proposed strategies. Family goals might not include therapy.

In addition, examination of the behaviors of the professionals who distress families through their interviews is needed to determine if their interactions are commensurate with community standards of ethics, not merely the mental health professional's interpretation of those standards. Such a review is rarely performed in a balanced manner. Most reasonable people would find the way in which the families were treated in both incidents as unreasonable. One can hardly imagine a family visiting a son or daughter in the intensive care unit of a general hospital to be confronted by 11 professionals and a television crew waiting to interview a family in crisis about sensitive, private information without their consent. Nor would one expect families visiting their relatives recovering from a diabetic coma to be treated in a similar way. These confrontations by staff are often faced by families of the seriously mentally ill.

Don't common community expressions of behaviors that govern how professionals and visitors relate in hospitals also apply to psychiatric settings? Wouldn't the average person be equally as outraged as the families in the cases described when constitutional rights were so flagrantly violated by health professionals at a time of crisis? Why haven't the policies of hospitals protected families from such aversive interventions? Why haven't the professionals who are aware of such interventions objected to such procedures and advocated on behalf of such families? Why haven't professional organizations addressed the ways in which many families have been mistreated in psychiatric facilities (Appleton 1974)? What has happened to society to permit such unethical practices with families in crisis? Why do families allow themselves to be treated so poorly by professionals? It is not possible to answer all the questions posed. If professionals are to continue to regulate their practices with families, the questions must be addressed by them. Families should press for answers soon, and they should develop their own strategies for change. Such a proposal is described at the end of this chapter.

WHY DO FAMILIES ALLOW THEMSELVES TO BE MISTREATED IN FAMILY INTERVIEWS?

It is not easy to discharge professionals because often the patient continues to need attention and care from them. It is not possible in such a crisis to move to another hospital. For example, Mrs. Jones, the mother cited in the second incident, continued to meet the psychiatrist in family therapy despite her anger at the way she was treated at the interview described. She reluctantly continued to see the psychiatrist because her daughter was still in the hospital and the mother had been informed that she was expected to participate in treatment. The mother feared retribution from the staff if she did not comply with treatment expectations. Mrs. Jones indicated that she no longer trusted the psychiatrist. She did report the incident to the psychiatrist's superior, who supported the young psychiatrist's actions.

After a formal complaint to the director, Mrs. Jones perceived that the staff on the unit where her daughter was hospitalized responded to her daughter and herself differently. The daughter's ward privileges were reduced, and she was no longer permitted to represent the unit at hospital-wide meetings, an activity of considerable importance to her. The staff encouraged others to discuss more openly and frequently the negative behavior displayed by the patient in ward meetings without protection or support from the staff. Emotional support from staff toward the patient was diminished as revealed in changes in documentation in the medical record. Visiting privileges for the mother were stopped and continued only after the mother agreed to continue in family therapy with the same therapist who had mistreated her at the family session described.

Many families anticipate this form of retribution from staff and will suffer silently rather than risk further discomfort for the hospitalized relative. Policies, regulations, and laws prohibiting this kind of practice by some professionals must be initiated to protect the rights of families to informed consent, dignity, and privacy. Families find these planned strategic practices of interviewing techniques without informed consent offensive, aversive, and distressing. Such practices are frequently discussed at NAMI meetings.

SANCTION FOR PROFESSIONALS TO GAIN COMPLIANCE FOR FAMILY INTERVIEWS

Incidents similar to the two described earlier even appear in professional publications without disclaimers from journal editors about the manner in which families are treated by professionals. Van Trommel (1984) described the reactions of a family who had not been asked if they would consent to a videotaped interview and agree to having others view them during the family session until the interview was to occur. This does not constitute informed consent because a timely disclosure of all facts, including potential risks, was not provided. Efforts were used by the professionals, particularly the psychiatrist, to gain family consent for the videotaping of the family interview by refusing to provide consultation to the parents regarding their son's illness if refusal to allow videotaping of the procedure occurred. Consultation from a psychiatrist was the reason the family was present.

Another article, by Hsia and Herman (1985), cited the importance of having families reinforce psychiatric treatment for relatives who were mentally impaired and unable to work. Their disability claims required periodic reevaluation from mental health professionals. The authors claimed that to engage the resistant patients in treatment, their families should be required to bring them to therapy sessions scheduled at 7:00 A.M. or at a similar inconvenient time. Patient or family noncompliance in treatment could result in professionals' withholding support for entitlement applications or continuations among the mentally ill persons. No disclaimer from the editor appeared with the article. Interestingly, family advocates were among the most aggressive in gaining increased money from the state legislature to support such community-based programs.

Other methods of gaining family treatment compliance appear in the professional literature. Strategies to use with such families are pervasive, often coercive, and underscore the problems faced by many consumers interacting with staff in mental health care delivery systems (Howe 1985; anonymous personal communications at AMI of Baltimore, Maryland, June 1983, April 1984, June 1985, and March 1986). Harbin (1982) described methods to use as a last resort when "rational persuasion" failed in working with families appearing to be resistant to family therapy. Some of the suggestions extended could be viewed as coercive and/or threatening if therapists used them in their work with families. Later, Harbin clarified the intent of that section of his book by emphasizing that the focus was not merely to engage the families in family therapy as an end point but to mobilize needed and active family support for a fragile or treatment-resistant patient. As a result of additional experience and feedback from family and consumer groups, such as NAMI chapters, Harbin has revised his thinking and recommendations about how to approach "resistant families" with chronically mentally ill relatives: strategies aimed at reducing patient noncompliance with treatment should be targeted toward the patient, and nonintrusive collaboration with families should be encouraged (H. Harbin, personal communication, 27 March 1986, Baltimore, Maryland).

Misleading assumptions about families do little to create useful interpersonal relations among staff and patients' relatives. The implications of forced family involvement in treatment, if carried to a logical conclusion, are to assume that the family, rather than the patient, is ill. Pejorative attitudes held by staff and actualized as treatment plans for families who have goals that are different from those of the treatment team could result in escalating family-staff conflict. Once begun, such conflicts are difficult to resolve (Harbin 1982). Efforts to prevent such dissonance should focus on methods to elicit family cooperation in the patient's rehabilitation plan based on an individualized assessment of all members' needs and goals (H. Harbin, personal communication, 27 March 1986, Baltimore, Maryland).

Families do not necessarily delegate to professionals all decisions affecting their role with their relatives when admission to a psychiatric hospital occurs. As Terkelsen (1983) suggested, resistant families may be products of a therapist's theoretical bias in viewing the family's role in the etiology of the illness. Often, professionals base practices on those psychogenic orientations. Perhaps in covert ways the therapist may communicate negative feelings or attitudes to families concerning a theoretical bias through his or her interviewing style. If premature discharge occurs, the patient could be denied active psychiatric treatment and the family could be placed in the position of caring for an actively psychotic individual without proper resources in the community. Even if the treatment team does not execute their overt or covert threat, it could terminate communication between the family and the team. Such threats are likely to destroy the mutual trust that is the foundation of any therapeutic alliance. At worst, it may contribute to a split between the patient and the family at a time when emotional, financial, and other forms of support are greatly needed by the mentally ill relative.

Torrey (1977) has referred to this type of distress as iatrogenic and wrote a satirical fantasy about a hypothetical class-action suit against professionals using such practices. However, iatrogenic distress is semantically incorrect, because it means distress created by a physician. The kind of distress created by professionals in the incidents described here are somewhat different because the discomfort caused was created by professionals from various disciplines who apparently had the sanction of the administration. This type of distress is referred to as *hygosystogenic*.

Hygosystogenic Distress

Hygosystogenic disorders or distress are induced by the health care team charged with caring for the patient and the family and are distinct from iatrogenic disorders, which are similar but caused by the physician. In this chapter, the term is used to describe the attitudes, injudicious remarks, and other actions or practices by the mental health care team that create distress in the patient or the patient's family. An assumption is made that the attitudes or actions are either outside the normal realm of practice, suggest aversive stereotyping of the recipients of the care, lack scientific merit from controlled studies, or are marginally acceptable practices that pose ethical and legal concerns between the professional care giver and the consumers of care.

Hygosystogenia means to become ill or distressed through the actions, attitudes, or practices of the health care team. Hygosystogenic illnesses can develop as a result of aversive experiences with health professionals regardless of the disorder or illness expressed by consumers. However, the term was coined as a result of extremely distressing practices of mental health professionals who unnecessarily increased the suffering of families through their transactions and/or interviewing styles.

Hygosystogenia is derived from three Greek words. *Hygo* is derived from Hygiea, who is personified as the goddess of health. The word refers to health medicine, cure, or soundness of body. *Systausis* refers to a guardianship, an alliance, in care. Hence, the concept involving the team of caretakers evolved. The word *gignomal* is translated as "to become" and is a common medical suffix.

The incidents involving Jane Doe and the Jones family illustrate how hygosystogenic distresses are created by the psychiatric team. Such distress is more complex than iatrogenic illnesses because a group of professionals—the team—caused the aversive psychological symptoms among the victims and these adverse behaviors of the professionals toward the parents were planned by the staff and were not merely the result of error or poor judgment of one individual, as would be the case in an iatrogenic etiology. The logical inference to be drawn is that such professional actions, which resulted in the family members' invasion of privacy and subsequent distress, had administrative and professional approval. To address such practices places more excessive demands on the victims than would occur if only one individual committed the error without the sanction of the staff or other groups.

DIRECTIONS FOR CHANGE

Persons involved in the distressing incident and the time, date, and location of the interview in question should be noted. Informing advocates about the incident and requesting assistance in addressing the distressing aspects of the situation are indicated because retribution from staff for formal complaints about their services is a possibility. It is likely that retribution will be less if an advocate outside the organization is involved, particularly if the organization has a large number of members who support the issue in question and have political power. Advocates employed by the organization are of little value in situations like those described in this chapter because the incidents could not have occurred without the sanction of the administration and the professional community. Hence, little assistance is to be expected from those employed by the hospital, thus supporting the need to develop a strong external change mechanism that includes guidelines, regulations, and consumer protection laws for families to ensure that informed consent, privacy, and community standards of conduct among professionals occur. Guidelines for professionals when interviewing families are offered in Table 1.

Families have an important role to play in stopping these unethical and often illegal practices by some professionals. Families should be encouraged to file grievances at the hospital where the incident occurred, with the proviso that a person outside the organization will monitor the family's perception of care rendered after registration of

Table 1. Guidelines to ensure informed consent when interviewing families

---

- Introduce yourself and inform the family members of your credentials for working with families, including academic qualifications, experience, and years of service with chronic populations.
- Inform the family of your theoretical orientation in working with families and why your requests of them should be considered.
- Explicitly state your goals and objectives for the proposed sessions.
- Ask families what their goals are from the mental health professionals. Be sure to obtain objectives from each family member to determine if your goals are congruent with the proposed participants' objectives.
- Develop an explicit and written working agreement with the family.
- Have a written informed consent form to be signed by all family members willing to participate in any electronic taping or procedures in which trainees are requested to observe. Families do not consider educating professionals to be their primary goal; they want assistance from providers. If families choose to reject the offer, honor their decision.

  - Ask the family (do not merely inform them) at least 1 week in advance if you wish to videotape, audiotape, or have observers present. Make clear your purpose in the use of electronic taping and observation and place the objectives in writing.
  - Include the number, types of professionals, and levels of training of the observers. Specify if nonprofessionals will be present or will have access to the tapes.
  - Indicate how the tapes will be stored to protect the privacy of the family members and how the names will be erased to provide anonymity.
  - Indicate how the tapes are intended to be used.
  - Families should be encouraged to seek legal counsel in regard to consent for videotaping in particular. Families should stipulate on the informed consent form any limits they wish to place on the viewing or dissemination of such materials. Clear distinctions should be made between use of tapes for *supervision* of the treating clinician and *training* of clinicians in other settings (Christine McGill, personal communication, 26 February 1986, Rockville, Maryland).
  - Families should have the opportunity to view taped materials after the fact.
  - After consenting to taping, families should have the right to withdraw their consent or request deletion of any objectionable material (Christine McGill, personal communication, 26 February 1986, Rockville, Maryland).

- Inform the family of potential risks of such behavioral interventions, which may include an increase in distress, loss of self-esteem, and the development of a sense of powerlessness.

continued

Table 1. Guidelines to ensure informed consent when
interviewing families *(continued)*

- A written statement in the informed consent form should indicate that
  if the family refuses to participate in the form of interviews proposed,
  the relative's treatment or privileges or the family's visiting rights will
  not be adversely affected.
- Do not coerce the family to engage in the interviews by threatening
  premature discharge of the relative from the hospital for noncompliance in family sessions. The parents are consenting adults.
- Do not coerce the family to engage in family interviews by threatening
  withdrawal of entitlements.
- If the family changes their decision to participate in the family sessions
  after attending a few sessions, honor their decision. Often families
  consent to sessions without fully understanding the procedures.
  Examine the therapeutic style of the professional to determine possible
  reasons for the family's termination. Referral to a person practicing
  supportive family counseling (Bernheim and Lehman 1982), a family
  education group (Hatfield 1983), or a family support group (NAMI)
  may be indicated.
- Provide in-service education programs for all professionals working
  with families on the impact of a serious mental illness from the family
  perspective, using family publications and families as educators. In
  addition, programs on ethical issues raised in family interviews should
  be addressed through continuing education programs (Margolin 1982;
  Hare-Mustin 1980; Terkelsen 1983; Lefley 1988).

---

the complaint. Actively working to address the mistreatment may help
to restore a sense of power and esteem to family members. Their
actions may help to prevent hygosystogenic distress for other families
in crisis, as occurred in the Doe case. In addition, families should be
informed of their right to file a complaint with the Joint Commission
on Accreditation of Health Care Organizations (JCAHO) for violations of their privacy and for failure of staff to provide the full implications of informed consent to them. Public hearings with JCAHO
surveyors are possible at a subsequently scheduled site visit for accreditation of the hospital. Such requests must be made in advance
of the visit (JCAHO 1985). The procedures for requesting such a
hearing are described in the NAMI consumer guide (Hatfield 1985).

Families may also wish to file a complaint with the professional
organization that licensed the provider committing the infraction.
This could initiate an investigation of the professional performance
of the staff member, because professionals have a code of ethics that
governs practice. It is unlikely that professionals employed by the
hospital where the staff committed the untoward actions are likely to

assertively elicit formal complaints or grievances from families because of possible retribution from administration, even though the professionals may empathize with the plight of these families. These facts mandate the creation of family advocates outside of the treatment facility or agency to assertively assist the family in the complex issues associated with staff-family conflicts. Again, the need for guidelines and consumer protection laws to regulate the professional's behavior for the purpose of protecting families from hygosystogenic distress and to ensure that their rights to informed consent and privacy are implemented is evidenced. Families or their representatives must consider strategic plans to stop these forms of mistreatment by mental health professionals.

Curriculum Content for Mental Health Professionals

Families' rights to informed consent and privacy in regard to interviews with staff in mental health care settings have implications for the preparation of future professionals and the formation of a system to address the unethical and legal issues impacting on some family members as they interact with the mental health care delivery system. The curriculum issues in education as professionals are socialized to their future roles with families must be examined.

The content and aims of educational programs have traditionally involved five basic orientations to the curriculum: 1) to foster the development of the student's cognitive processes; 2) to promote intellectual growth of the student in those matters worthy of study; 3) to discover personal relevance; 4) to underscore the importance of serving the interests of society; and 5) to relate the results of the educational program to the means for obtaining the education, i.e., to evaluate the program of study. According to Eisner (1982), the five orientations provide a way of rationalizing what schools teach and are referred to as the explicit curriculum. Syllabi reflect the content of the explicit curriculum.

Eisner (1982) claims that schools teach much more than the overt explicit curriculum. The "hidden," or implicit, curriculum has tremendous sociological and psychological impact and tends to socialize students to a set of expectations that some argue are more powerful and persistent than what is intentionally taught in the explicit curriculum. The implicit curriculum of a school is conveyed to students covertly by representatives of the school, usually through role models. The therapists' behavior toward the Doe and the Jones families could be inferred to evolve from the implicit curriculum as suggested by the lack of preparation of the parents for the interview by the teachers. Other professionals may imitate these approaches because the teachers are distinguished role models. What was taught to the student observers is speculative; yet the unethical professional practices had tremendous impact on the families involved and created the hygosystogenic distress.

However, the students are also influenced by what schools do not teach. This is referred to as the null curriculum. Because omissions in educational preparation limit perspectives and increase biases for appraising evidence and making sound professional judgments, the null curriculum has a tremendous impact on clinical practice. Graduates of programs in which critical material is lacking may espouse a parochial perspective or offer simplistic solutions to complex problems through naïveté or ignorance. The result is that consumers of services rendered by those providers do not receive optimal care. One can speculate that the professionals involved in the incidents described earlier were the products of educational programs in which ethical aspects of professional behavior toward families were lacking and, hence, were part of the null curriculum. In addition, legal implications of professional practice and its relationship to families can be inferred to be deficits in the professional preparation of those staff cited in the Doe and the Jones incidents. The obvious implications of these findings, based on the analysis of the cases cited and the apparent effective in-service approach by staff in the hospital regarding the Doe case, are to place ethical and legal aspects of professional transactions with families in the explicit curriculum of all professional training programs. The material should be realistic and repeatedly reinforced by prestigious role models to allow assimilation into the professional's practice repertoire with families. Some recommendations for the explicit curriculum follow.

1. Understanding the impact of a major mental illness on a valued relative from the family's perspective should be required of all persons prepared to work with the seriously mentally ill (Lefley 1988).
2. Professional trainees should be observers at family support group meetings over sufficient time to learn alternatives to therapy for working with such families.
3. Family education programs similar to the type offered by Hatfield (1983) should be offered to professionals in understanding the impact of the relative's illness (Harbin 1985; since 1982, the Mental Hygiene Administration has funded and promoted statewide family education sessions and publications. The objectives are to inform, support, and decrease some of the burden faced by families of the seriously mentally ill.). Professionals need to be taught such educational and group-process strategies, because the ap-

proaches differ from a therapy model, and must consider the families as adult learners.

4. Guidelines for interviewing families should address the goals of the families, not merely the objectives as interpreted by professionals. This is an important function because evidence exists that families and professionals often have different perceptions of need (Spaniol et al. 1984) and hold different views of what bothers families about caring for a mentally ill relative (McElroy 1987).

5. Professionals should gain an understanding of the families' beliefs about what they think caused the illness. It is especially important to provide current scientific information on this topic because studies have shown that people take responsibility for causing illnesses affecting themselves or their relatives regardless of the disease (Mabry 1964; Lowery and Jacobsen 1985). These attributions of causality can often be a source of unnecessary guilt.

6. The timing of interventions with families should be taught to new professionals. Professionals should refrain from always doing a genogram or focusing on the family communication patterns early in their involvement with families. These behaviors among professionals tend to suggest that something about the family's behavioral style or interpersonal relationships caused the illness or relapse and can lead to guilt or hygosystogenic distress. Gathering such data needs to be considered only after a good relationship between the family and staff has been successfully established.

7. The cyclic chronic mental illnesses often require planning for relapse and rehospitalization. Proper preparation and planning by informed, sensitive professionals who will provide continuity of care are essential. Helping families and patients to cope with such treatment plans without feeling a sense of failure is essential.

8. Videotapes of families being interviewed by professionals who have violated their ethical and human rights should be shown in training programs to stimulate discussion to learn from these failures (Coleman 1985). Families, lawyers, mental health professionals, and experts on medical ethics should comprise panels, react to such tapes, and offer solutions to these practices.

The following changes for the mental health care delivery system are suggested to ensure that informed consent and privacy are guaranteed to all families.

1. Informed consent should be required on all behavioral interventions that are applied to families.

2. Guidelines for interviewing family members should be required.

3. Regulations should eventually be developed that would require accreditation groups to examine policies, procedures, and medical records of family treatment.
4. Disclosure of accreditation reports on psychiatric facilities should be available to the public.
5. Consumer protection laws should be developed to ensure compliance with guidelines created by family advocates.
6. Access to persons with expertise on medical ethics should be available for professionals when disagreements about treatments affecting families occur between family and staff.
7. A think-tank organization independent of the mental health care delivery system is needed to study policies and practices affecting families in psychiatric facilities. The format of such a group would include consensus workshops where position papers on a topic are developed by experts, public discussions occur, and the ensuing suggestions are assimilated in the final recommendations made by the members.

Until such changes occur, families of the seriously mentally ill must carefully consider the first rule of consumerism as they relate to representatives of the mental health care delivery system—*caveat emptor*, "the buyer beware."

REFERENCES

American Medical Association: Principles of Medical Ethics of the American Medical Association. Chicago, IL, American Medical Association, 1954

Anderson C, Stewart S: Mastering Resistance: A Practical Guide to Family Therapy. New York, Guilford, 1983

Annotated Code of Maryland, HG §§ 4-301–303, 81–85; HO § 14–504 (1982)

Appleton WS: Mistreatment of patients' families by psychiatrists. Am J Psychiatry 22:665–667, 1974

Beane v McMullen, 265 Md 585, 291 A2d 37 (1972)

Bernheim KF, Lehman AF: Teaching mental health trainees to work with families of the chronic mentally ill. Hosp Community Psychiatry 46:1109–1111, 1985

Breggin PR: Electroshock. New York, Springer, 1979

Coleman SB: Failures in Family Therapy. New York, Guilford, 1985

Eisner E: Cognition and Curriculum: A Basis for Deciding What to Teach. White Plains, NY, Longman, 1982

Harbin H: Family treatment of the psychiatric patient, in Psychiatric Hospital and the Family. New York, SP Medical & Scientific Books, 1982

Harbin H: Maryland Department of Health and Mental Hygiene budget request and report (monographed report). Baltimore, MD, state of Maryland, 1985

Hare-Mustin RT: Family therapy may be dangerous for your health. Professional Psychology 11:935–938, 1980

Hare-Mustin RT, Marecek J, Kaplan AG, et al: Rights of clients, responsibilities of therapists. Am Psychol 34:3–16, 1979

Hatfield AB: Coping With Mental Illness in the Family: The Family Guide. Baltimore, Mental Hygiene Administration of Maryland, 1983

Hatfield AB: Consumer Guide for Mental Health Service. Arlington, VA, National Alliance for the Mentally Ill, 1985

Hollander v Lubow, 277 Md 47, 351 A2d 421

Howe C: Responding to families of mentally ill children and youth. Paper presented at the 23rd annual Child Psychiatry Forum, Richmond, VA, May 1985

Hsia H, Herman R: Strategies in working with chronically unemployed mental patients. Hosp Community Psychiatry 36:777–779, 1985

Joint Commission on Accreditation of Hospitals (JCAH): Accreditation Manual for Hospitals. Chicago, IL, JCAH, 1985

Lefley HP: Training professionals to work with families of chronic patients. Community Ment Health J 24:338–357, 1988

Lowery BJ, Jacobsen BS: Attributional analysis of chronic illness outcomes. Nurs Res 34:82–88, 1985

Mabry JH: Lay concepts of etiology. J Chronic Dis 17:371–386, 1964

McElroy E: Families and mental health professionals march to the beat of a different drummer, in Families as Caregivers. Edited by Lefley H, Hatfield A. New York, Guilford, 1987

Margolin G: Ethical and legal considerations in marital and family therapy. Am Psychol 37:788–801, 1982

Plotkin R: Limiting the therapeutic orgy: mental patients' right to refuse treatment. Northwestern University Law Review 72:461–525, 1977

Prosser WL, Keeton WP: The Law of Tort, 5th Edition. St. Paul, MN, West, 1985, pp 807–808

Reinstatement Second, Torts, Tentative Draft No 21, § 652 (1975)

Ruben HL, Ruben D: Confidentiality and privileged communications: the psychotherapeutic relationship revisited. Medical Annals of the District of Columbia 41:364–368, 1972

Shaw v Glickman, 45 Md App 718, 415 A2d 625 (June 13, 1980)

Slovenko R, Udin GL: Psychiatry, Confidentiality, and Privileged Communication. Springfield, IL, Charles C Thomas, 1966

Spaniol L, Jung H, Zipple AM, et al: Families as a Central Resource in the Rehabilitation of the Severely Psychiatrically Disabled: Report of a National Survey. Boston, MA, Boston University, 1983

Terkelsen KG: Schizophrenia and the family: adverse effects of family therapy. Fam Process 22:191–200, 1983

Torrey EF: A fantasy trial about a real issue. Psychology Today 10:24, 1977

Van Trommel MJ: A consultation method addressing the therapist-family system. Fam Process 22:469–480, 1984

Walsh M: Schizophrenia: Straight Talk for Families and Friends. New York, William Morrow, 1985

Informed Consent, Confidentiality, and Contracting

Leroy Spaniol, Ph.D.

The onset of mental illness in a family member creates a severe crisis for the whole family. In addition to the considerable distress caused by the illness itself, families feel bruised and frustrated by a mental health system that they feel lacks the resources, the competence, and the sensitivity to assist them in this very tragic human event (Lefley 1989). Dr. McElroy's chapter is an important contribution to creating awareness of the concerns of families in crisis, the need for the protection of the basic human rights of family members, and how the attitudes and practices of some mental health professionals violate these rights and add to the distress of families.

The initial focus of the chapter is on issues of informed consent and confidentiality. It might be beneficial to distinguish between these two concepts, because they are not equivalent. The purpose of informed consent is to protect the rights, in general, of humans. Confidentiality refers to the protection of one of those rights, the right to privacy. Informed consent usually includes the right of confidentiality as one of the protected rights. The concerns of Dr. McElroy and the concept of informed consent go beyond privacy to include other rights such as protection from psychological abuse and protection from denial of service.

The protection of rights is clearly a concern of family members. It is also a major concern of consumers and mental health professionals. All parties share concerns for individual rights, but often their

195

perspectives or beliefs concerning when, how, and which rights to protect differ. For example, Dr. McElroy clearly identifies families' concerns about the lack of informed consent for family members in their relationships with professionals. Yet, families are also concerned about the limits the patient's right to privacy puts on the information available to families about what is happening to their mentally ill family member. Patients are concerned about information on their disability and progress being made available to individuals outside the immediate treatment team, including family members. Mental health professionals struggle with what at times appear to be the benefits and at times the constraints that patients' rights to privacy put on communications with families. Given the increasing number of parties wanting to have some say in decisions affecting a person with a severe mental illness, given the presence, at times, of negative beliefs and attitudes of these parties toward one another, and given the possibility of the current processes by which we arrive at our decisions seriously bruising one or more of these parties, it is critical that we increase our awareness, respect, and protection of the rights, wants, and roles that these various parties require.

The immediate focus of Dr. McElroy's chapter is on protecting the rights of families in the interviewing process. She discussed the potential risks to family members and provided examples of injury that she felt have occurred to family members. Dr. McElroy proposed informed consent as one practical solution to protecting family rights. The basic components of informed consent include

1. Stating the purpose and goals of the process
2. Stating the uses of the information generated by the process
3. Identifying how the information will be stored
4. Identifying potential risks of the process
5. Indicating that the decision to participate or not to participate will not influence future decisions regarding the person agreeing to the process
6. Indicating freedom of the person agreeing to the process to discontinue or limit participation at any time
7. Indicating the limits of anonymity and confidentiality

Dr. McElroy added to the above list a number of other protections specific to contacts with family members. There are numerous problems in utilizing informed consent as the model for clarifying the relationship between the family and the mental health professional. Informed consent does not tend to be a negotiating process. The informed consent form is presented as a given that the person can either accept or reject. Families clearly are not satisfied with the parameters of the current family-professional relationship. Families want to be part of the process by which these parameters are defined; they do not want to accept them as givens.

Informed consent also assumes that the professional knows best how to protect the parties involved. Dr. McElroy's comments and the experiences of many family members suggest that this may not necessarily be the case. Informed consent assumes a relationship that is unequal. The professional determines the parameters, and the person accepts or rejects them. Family members consider themselves to be equals of mental health professionals and do not want to be treated as patients or "subjects." Informed consent tends to limit itself to several core protections without maintaining flexibility around those protections or considering the addition of new protections as the situation demands them. Family-professional relationships require flexibility and negotiation because of the inherent ambiguity of the nature of the disability and the processes by which we hope to heal it. Finally, informed consent focuses primarily on the protection of rights, whereas families are also concerned about the nature of the family-professional relationship and how this can be clarified in ways that promote sensitivity and communication and enhance the rehabilitation for their disabled family member.

Perhaps an alternative model to informed consent might be that of a contract. A contract implies equality, competence of contractors, mutual consent, a negotiation of specifics, the involvement of both parties in the processes by which the contract is arrived at, specific roles, specific effort, and specific goals. A model for a contractual arrangement between the family and a mental health system or practitioner might include the following:

1. Mutual consent
   - Negotiation of the purpose and goals of the process by all parties
   - Negotiation of uses of information generated by the treatment process
   - Negotiation of where information will be stored
   - Negotiation of potential risks for all parties
   - Negotiation of how future decisions regarding all parties will be influenced by the decision of one or more of the parties to participate or not to participate
   - Negotiation of the consequences for limiting or terminating participation in the process for all parties
   - Negotiation of the roles and efforts of all parties
   - Negotiation of the boundaries of anonymity and confidentiality

2. Mutual acceptance
   - All parties agree to the conditions they have mutually nego-
     tiated.
   - When any party wishes to change the conditions, a renegotia-
     tion will occur.

There are some problems and some advantages to a contracting
arrangement between families and professionals. Contracting takes
time and effort. Professionals and families are already quite overwhelmed by their tasks. The solution for the professional is to start
with one family and to be open to listening and negotiating with that
family. As professionals begin to work this way with families, they will
begin to increase their confidence and sense of competence in the
process. Professionals may also find that working cooperatively with
families may actually create more time for other professional activities.
Families can be an important resource and source of support in the
rehabilitation of their disabled family member. Some professionals
may feel there is little supervisory or peer support for a contracting
approach with families. It is difficult being a pioneer. If the professional feels personally committed and is willing to communicate his
or her beliefs and attitudes to supervisors and peers, the professional
may find more support than he or she thought was there. Again,
starting with a few families will provide an experiential basis for advocating a more cooperative approach with families.

One of the advantages of the contracting approach is its simplicity.
It can be learned by staff and by families with a limited amount of
training or orientation. It also helps to avoid the potential for "bruising" one another. Contracting increases sensitivity and communication among all involved parties. Contracting can also help to avoid
the "crises orientation" of some mental health practices and of some
families' relationship with their disabled family member. Contracting
ensures that most potential problems will receive help in a predictable
way. People can learn to count on the resources that are available.
Contracting also facilitates the monitoring of the effectiveness of the
agreed-on process. The focus can shift from blaming one another for
the breakdown of the process to trying to understand what went
wrong and how each person can work together to fix it. Finally, working together in a mutually agreed-on way by its very nature seems to
increase the likelihood of positive outcome.

Dr. McElroy's final comments are on the education of mental
health professionals. The points she makes are well worth attending
to and should be included in any curriculum on families of the mentally ill for professionals. There are several concerns I would like to
add to her suggested curriculum. The first is the need to increase

professional awareness of the process of family adjustment to the crises of mental illness in a family member. Families experience a process that includes shock, denial, anger, grief, acceptance, and advocacy (Tessler et al. 1987). Those familiar with the literature on families of the mentally retarded or the physically disabled will readily recognize this process (Power and Dell Orto 1980). Information on what is happening to families as they react and attempt to cope with a family member with a severe mental illness can help sensitize mental health professionals to what families are experiencing. Professionals need to understand the human dimension of what is happening to families and the information, support, and skills that families need to move from a reactive to a more advocacy-oriented mode. In addition, professionals need to understand the possibilities and the limits of their ability to help families at each stage of the families' adjustment and coping. The possibilities include the roles that professionals can play, such as that of a resource or a teacher. The limits include the needs that families have for their own support and advocacy process with other families, independent of professional supervision.

An additional curriculum concern is addressing the need for professionals to be aware of the processes they go through as they confront their own attitudes and beliefs concerning families of the mentally ill. Professionals experience the same shock, denial, anger, grief, acceptance, and advocacy that families experience. In fact, these are universal human experiences associated with undergoing any significant change in our lives. Trainers need to understand this process because this new curriculum on families will threaten and challenge the attitudes and beliefs of mental health practitioners. Unless this underlying process is acknowledged and dealt with in the training itself, trainers run the risk of building up a new repertoire of knowledge without significantly affecting the attitudes and beliefs of the trainees.

Because of the critical needs to impact on the attitudes and beliefs of mental health practitioners, it is especially important to include family members in the planning, implementation, and evaluation of any training intervention with professionals. Attitudes and beliefs are influenced most profoundly by significant experiences. It is the experience of family members as cotrainers, over time, plus the information that professional trainers can teach, that will most likely lead to important changes in professional attitudes and beliefs. The experience with family members must be substantive. Brief contact, such as in a periodic presentation by a family member, will not allow professionals to adequately undergo their own process of adjustment to working with families in new ways and may in fact reinforce denial and increase negative attitudes. Mental health professionals need to acquire new information about families, and they need to learn to feel comfortable with this new information. Both the learning of information and the acquisition of "comfort" are essential ingredients of any training intervention.

Finally, there is a need for new models for understanding the experience of families of the mentally ill, family-professional relationships, and the role of the family in the rehabilitation of their psychiatrically disabled family member. The models and meanings that professionals currently bring to their relationships with families are no longer valid. Professionals need new ways to understand families. It is not enough to say that what is currently believed is no longer adequate. We must be ready to present new models and meanings for consideration to professionals while they are going through their own changes in beliefs and attitudes. We must be clear about what is no longer adequate or acceptable, and we must present some viable options.

REFERENCES

Lefley HP: Family burden and family stigma in major mental illness. Am Psychol 44:556–560, 1989

Power P, Dell Orto A: Role of the family in the rehabilitation of the physically disabled. Baltimore, MD, University Park Press, 1980

Tessler RC, Killian LM, Gubman G: Stages in family response to mental illness: an ideal type. Psychosocial Rehabilitation Journal 10:3–16, 1987

Chapter 7

Promoting Institutional Acceptance of New Paradigms: An Approach to the Professional Schools

Gerda Cohen, A.C.S.W.
Kenneth G. Terkelsen, M.D.

Previous contributors have documented the need for a new paradigm for relations between families of the mentally ill and mental health professionals. In this chapter, we address the task of making contact with faculty in the graduate professional schools and influencing what they communicate to their students about families of the long-term mentally ill.

The professional schools, more than any other institutional setting within the mental health scene, shape the young professional's core attitudes toward self and client. Those attitudes are the bedrock on which the professional's future development takes place. When a student learns to regard families as toxic forces for the mentally ill and adversaries in the treatment process, it is likely that the student will go on to acquire knowledge and skills that demonstrate over and over that families are noxious and adversarial. By contrast, the student whose early experiences suggest that families make a contribution to the healing process and that relatives, along with the patient, suffer under the impact of the illness will more than likely seek information and skills that confirm the family's helpfulness and reveal the relative's agony.

In another sense, we are moving beyond the previous chapters in this book, centering less on what is to be taught and more on the process of gaining access to a school and supporting faculty efforts to bring about their own paradigm shift. We will describe what we have done in classrooms—what we have said and how—but the description throughout will be in the service of taking the reader on a tour of the steps leading the school in question to permanently own the spirit that we brought to students during our brief visits. In this chapter, then, we are attempting to elucidate how the deep structure of the encounter between a team from the Alliance for the Mentally Ill (AMI) and the students and faculty whom we have visited catalyzes institutional movement toward enabling clinical paradigms.

In the description that follows, we will attempt to identify the relevant general principles informing each crucial aspect of the process and then to describe specific steps we took to actualize those principles. In truth, we were often acting on instinct in this project and could abstract the general principles only later and with some distance from the intensity and immediacy of visits to the school. It should also be said at the outset that, although we have now gone through two teaching cycles in this school, we are not yet so confident in our evolving perspective to claim that it has generic applicability. We believe that substantial modification will occur as the basic methods we are elaborating are brought to different schools by other teams. We are surprised that our presence is making a difference in attitudes toward families and that we are greeted and valued by any members of the faculty at all. In the face of this acceptance, we have sought to vary the basic visit, taking risks in the service of discovering durable generic principles that could be applied in other settings.

DEVELOPING A BASE OF LEGITIMACY

During meetings of AMI of New York, we became aware that there were a number of AMI members in New York who, as relatives of mentally ill persons, were also mental health professionals. We reasoned that as persons with dual-experience backgrounds, we might be in an ideal position to make contact with graduate professional schools. We were not necessarily known as relatives of mentally ill persons, or as members of the AMI movement, within our own institutions. When we were, this knowledge did not automatically confer any extra authority on us in the eyes of our colleagues and students. (Indeed, we wondered whether the revelation of our unusual status might not lead to our being discredited rather than empowered to speak for the issues of families of the mentally ill.) Therefore, it seemed essential to create a base of organizational legitimacy within the AMI movement, a status that would be easily understood by the faculty and students we would encounter in the schools. We accomplished this by forming a committee to look into matters of curriculum and training in the professional schools, as an official part of the hierarchical structure of AMI of New York.

We, a clinical social worker (Cohen) and a psychiatrist (Terkelsen), having direct experience with schizophrenia in a family member, became the AMI team that would see the project through the first 2 years.

THE TEAM MODELS THE NEW PARADIGM

Early in our discussions, we took stock of our resources. We noted that together we could represent two kinds of teams: On the one hand, we were a relative and a mental health professional; on the other hand, we were a social worker and a psychiatrist. At both levels, we were interested in the welfare of families of the mentally ill and of mentally ill persons themselves. We saw that we could draw on both statuses and on both levels of interest in the work that would follow in the schools. When we wanted to convey the importance of teaching students to think of families as collaborators in work with the mentally ill, we would model that type of collaboration by approaching faculty and students as a family-and-professional team. When we wanted to highlight the scale of the movement embodied in AMI, we would represent ourselves as members of AMI of New York. Conversely, when we wanted to underscore the implications of our message for social work practice, we would become mental health clinicians with an interest in rehabilitation and education. Although much of this was done by intuition and in the moment, we believe that the flexibility accorded by our dual status as family members and as mental health professionals enhanced our authority within the schools. In retrospect, it occurred to us that the dual role we developed is not unlike the dual legitimacy of AMI members lobbying their legislators, who represent themselves both as relatives of the mentally ill and as constituents.

A SPECIAL KIND OF ADVOCACY

An additional feature of the work with the schools deserves mention here. We observed that many members of AMI of New York were evolving into capable, outspoken lobbyists for improved services. Typically, the task of confronting legislators and local and state officials in the mental health bureaucracy requires a capacity for vigorous, adversarial confrontation. We felt, however, that the approach to the schools required a radically different form of advocacy. Unlike public bureaucracies, schools do not have specific programmatic responsibilities and stated goals against which to measure the conduct of their task. Furthermore, professional faculty typically pride themselves on their independence of thought and invulnerability to public pressure in the pursuit of their mission. Therefore, it seemed imperative to approach the schools less as lobbyists and more as invited guests. Instead of hammering away at the deans of the schools, we would attempt to get ourselves invited to interact with the faculty as colleagues. Instead of challenging the faculty for teaching the old paradigm, we would show them how to teach the new paradigm. And instead of scolding students for the sins of their elders, we would give them an example of the new paradigm in practice. We would become emissaries for the kind of relations between professionals and relatives that we knew the schools must learn to foster.

We make note of this particular orientation here because some might think that advocacy this gentle and this collaborative is akin to selling out and that we were too interested in being liked by the faculty. In point of fact, because the faculties control access to students and decide what experiences are to be made available to students, the invitational approach was very much a part of the design for gaining access to the life of the school.

THE FIRST OVERTURE

As we considered which schools to make contact with, our first decision was to narrow the field to those that either of us could interface with on professional grounds. Thus, we considered schools of social work and psychiatric residency programs as the first candidates for our attention. Subsequently, we elected to center on the schools of social work for two reasons. First, we reasoned that this particular team would be accorded more respect a priori among social work faculty than among members of a department of psychiatry. Second, we believed the need for a new paradigm was more urgent among social workers. Within institutional settings, social workers are usually the family's primary contact point with the service in which a patient is treated. Third, we felt that social workers were less likely to be exposed to biological concepts of mental illness than were psychiatric residents. Finally, we believed between us that if social workers could be inspired to take work with this population and with their families seriously, social work as a profession would make a very significant contribution to the development of social, residential, and occupational environments in which the long-term mentally ill could live and regain access to meaningful involvements in the community.

Accordingly, in the spring of 1984, we wrote to the deans of several schools of social work in the metropolitan New York area, as follows:

> The ALLIANCE FOR THE MENTALLY ILL OF NEW YORK STATE is a coalition of 26 mutual family support and advocacy groups and an affiliate of the NATIONAL ALLIANCE FOR THE MENTALLY ILL. AMI aims to improve the quality of life of all people afflicted with chronic mental illness. AMI works toward securing better care and treatment in hospitals, better community services, increased funding for research, and toward empowering families to better cope with mental illness.
>
> As a result of the deinstitutionalization movement, two-thirds of the chronically mentally ill now live either in the family home or in residences nearby. Though families now assume a major role in the care and rehabilitation of these patients, professionals do little to assist them in shouldering this difficult responsibility.
>
> Moreover, the common belief that mental illness (especially schizophrenia) arises from family interaction sets up negative professional attitudes toward these families. By focusing on patterns of family interaction, professionals unwittingly increase guilt and foster forms of interaction that adversely affect the patient.
>
> AMI seeks to ensure that professional schools are preparing students to interact appropriately with families of the chronically mentally ill. Accordingly, AMI urges you to determine whether the present curriculum is in keeping with the needs of families of the chronically mentally ill. Through its Curriculum and Training Committee, AMI is prepared to work with the dean to develop learning experiences that provide the knowledge, skills, and attitudes required for work with the families of the mentally ill.

Our intention in this initial overture was to identify schools that were already close enough to the new paradigm to be able to see the need for and the value of dialogue with an AMI team.

HELP FROM WITHIN

When we first sent this letter to the deans of the New York schools of social work in the spring of 1984, we imagined we would be butting up against a nearly impenetrable wall of indifference or hostility in each and every school. Thus, we were surprised to receive an early response from George Braeger, dean of the Columbia University School of Social Work. That Dean Braeger remembered Cohen from their days in the school many years earlier may have been an important aspect of gaining entry and speaks strongly for the utility of finding people inside the school who are unusually accessible to the team's request for dialogue. In the case of Columbia, Dean Braeger's personal familiarity with Cohen, together with his knowledge (not stated in the letter) of Cohen's status as an alumnus of the school may have been the ties that afforded us access.

In our recent approaches, two other forms of a priori accessibility have become apparent. First, in a large school there are often several faculty who have personal experience with mental illness, or at least with significant behavioral disturbance, in a relative. These persons often remain silent within the school even though they have, by their personal experience, been brought to a full awareness of the need for changes in what the schools teach about mental illness and about the families of the mentally ill. They are silenced by their assessment that to become outspoken as individuals in their own schools would not by itself bring about any material change in what is taught. They require the backing of a reference group, which, until the appearance of the AMI team in the schools, has been nonexistent.

Second, we have encountered faculty who are taking a critical look at the old paradigm strictly on professional, methodological grounds and finding it lacking. Their faith in what they have been teaching has declined as they have come to realize that many methods in the domains of deinstitutionalization and family therapy have not yielded superior results for the patient population but have increased the family's care-giving burden and the impact of the illness on well relatives.

Whether through personal connections with members of the team or personal experience in the area of the team's work, or from professional skepticism about the old paradigm, we believe that an AMI team is most likely to have an initial favorable reception where inside support is available. As a result, we have tended increasingly to approach schools manifesting a priori recognition of the value of the team's potential contribution to the curriculum. We go when and where we are invited, developing a reputation as valued guests and then enlisting our newfound allies in one school to open doors in other schools that may have seemed uninterested or frankly unresponsive to our own overtures.

THE SCHOOL PICKS UP ON OUR INVITATION

Dean Braeger responded to our letter by inviting us to discuss the issues with him. He was receptive to our proposal that we give a presentation to the students, but he indicated that he could not be certain of wide support within the faculty. He emphasized that the faculty teach very nearly what they want to teach. We offered to meet with the whole faculty to dialogue on the issues of concern to us. Instead, in the aftermath of the first meeting, Dean Braeger approached one of the professors who he knew to have great sympathy for our cause.

OUR FIRST VISIT

Without hesitation, Dr. Renee Solomon invited us to give a workshop during one session of her second-year practicum course. She asked that we visit immediately after the sequence on the major mental illnesses. We later learned that Dr. Solomon had so strongly endorsed our visit to her students that we were talking to her entire class, even though the class met in the afternoon of the day before Thanksgiving. We asked Dr. Solomon to introduce us as representatives of AMI of New York. She spontaneously added Cohen's status as an alumnus of the school.

> After a warm introduction by Dr. Solomon, Cohen and Terkelsen proceeded to sit side by side in front of the students. While Terkelsen looked on, Cohen opened the 2-hour class by explaining the team's affiliation with AMI of New York. This entailed briefly describing what the AMI movement is, describing the National AMI, tracing the meteoric rise of local groups in the previous 5 years, linking this development to the shift from institutional care to community-based care, underscoring the increase in family burden, and alerting students to the fact that families are functioning as principal care givers for their ill relatives without guidance, without respite, and without acknowledgment of the critical role they are playing.

We were mindful at this juncture that we were invited guests and that Dr. Solomon had her own reasons for wanting her students to be exposed to our message. That is, although we were bringing a new message, we were there because among all the faculty, Dr. Solomon was already—to an unknown degree—an advocate for our position. We were also aware that, as useful as talking to this group of students might be, our central aim was to open a dialogue with the faculty through Dr. Solomon. Thus, it was imperative that we take a nonconfrontational orientation to the material, without at the same time diluting the necessary intensity of the message.

> Sharing from personal experience and drawing from experiences of friends in AMI, Cohen described what it is like for a family to cope with mental illness firsthand and day-to-day. Using the device of a guided fantasy, she asked the students to imagine what it would be like to send off a healthy, bright young man to college only to have him return in a state of acute disorganization some months later, hardly recognizable to the family; to imagine the exhaustive, frustrating search for professional help, made more difficult by the patient's unwillingness to collaborate in seeking help and repeated terminations from treatment. She asked the students to consider the family's

plight when one psychiatrist after another declines to sit with the family and explain what is happening, and when family therapists challenge their motivation vis-á-vis the patient with the notion that they need the child's illness to fill a void in their lives or even to save their marriage. Over and over, Cohen repeated the invitation to take the parent's part in listening to the story, and then in very even tones told of one frightening or discouraging or frustrating encounter after another. She deliberately emphasized that she and her husband were looking for understanding and support, information and guidance from the professionals in her son's life and how often they were turned away. To defuse the rising tension of this dialectic, she introduced an anecdote describing a late-night visit by one of the local town policemen. Her son was on the road. Her husband and friends were out looking for him. And she remained at home in her terror. Mindful of her agony, the policeman looked in on her, stopping for a cup of coffee and sharing the vigil with her for a few moments. She then turned the tenor of the story to more optimistic things, reporting that after some years of instability, her son was now fully employed and living with the woman of his choice. She recounted anecdotes she had heard from other families. She told of a young man who, after many years of total withdrawal and uncooperativeness, gave his mother a single rose on her birthday. In concluding her remarks, Cohen underscored the value she had found in listening to the experiences of other families going through similar difficulties and in this way pointed to the role of the local AMI chapters in providing emotional support for families. She emphasized that because of professional indifference these families had until recently been totally on their own in coping with the illness and the ill relative.

We anticipated that the intensely personal nature of this account would generate strong emotional responses among the students. Students would certainly have been swept into identifying with the position and the experience of the relative. There might also be, however, unknown degrees of guilt, confusion, or helplessness as students merged with one or another facet of the experience. We wanted to demonstrate to Dr. Solomon, and through her to the larger faculty, that a personal account could serve as the basis for effective attitudinal learning. Therefore, Cohen kept her remarks to 30 minutes, although it would have been easy to go on for another hour. We intended to search for student reactions, building a context in which it would be safe to dialogue on the issues raised by the account.

After her account, Cohen entertained questions. The students appeared delighted to hear a tale of plain human compassion and excited by the anecdotes of mutual aid given by AMI support groups. Of greatest interest was the interstate network of supportive services for wandering patients. Amid expressions of strong resonance with the experience, two students chose this moment to reveal that they also had personal experience with a mentally ill family member. These revelations, which would recur in other classroom encounters, served to further authenticate the validity and importance of our message for the students. Other questions, concerning what would have been a useful response from the professionals that Cohen had encountered, led directly into the second half of the workshop.

We knew that the strong emotional appeal of a personal account, especially one that was told in an organized manner and was laced with a measure of optimism, would create a condition of accessibility among students.

FROM ATTITUDES TO INFORMATION

However, the task of the faculty is to teach knowledge and skills as well as to communicate attitudes. So we came prepared to amplify the attitudinal learnings of Cohen's account with a distinctively academic presentation in the same universe of ideas given by Terkelsen. We assumed that to have maximal impact on a faculty that was, to an indeterminate extent, still involved with the old paradigm, we would have to offer an intellectual criticism of the old paradigm. It would not be enough to say that old-paradigm concepts are harmful to families; we would have to show the faculty, through the medium of talking to their students, that these ideas are not substantiated by careful empirical investigation. Additionally, we would have to offer a compelling alternative, which the faculty could absorb as the basis of their own future teaching in this area. Thus, when students asked Cohen what would have been a more useful response from the professionals she and other families had encountered, she turned the meeting over to Terkelsen, who undertook the academic phase of the workshop.

> Terkelsen addressed two major questions. First, he acknowledged that many of the students were probably wondering whatever became of the family interaction theories of schizophrenia. Second, he developed the basic concepts for the new-paradigm approach to work with families. In addressing the first question, Terkelsen reviewed the observable interactional phenomena that had led investigators of the 1940s and 1950s to hypothesize that family interaction might be making a contribution to the development of schizophrenia. Then he reviewed four generic ways of accounting for the co-occurrence of these family interaction phenomena with schizophrenia in an offspring. Type one theories posit that certain forms of family interaction produce a proneness for schizophrenic thought disorder. Type two theories posit that these same forms of family interaction are a response to certain aspects of the behavior of the schizophrenic patient. Type three theories suggest that genetically inherited disorders of attention may predispose to thought disorder in the patient and

simultaneously to certain types of unusual communicational behavior in other relatives. Type four theories posit that some of the unusual behavior seen in family meetings is the family's response to being observed by clinicians, especially if the clinicians have given evidence that they believe the family to have contributed to the development of the illness. Describing his own professional journey through this territory, Terkelsen spoke of his own early devotion to Type one theories and his growing skepticism, culminating in a crisis in confidence 5 years earlier, when he looked carefully at the empirical literature purporting to support Type one theories. He shared his own conclusion that at present there is no compelling empirical basis for preferring one type of explanation over any other and that, as a result, clinicians may not safely use Type one models in developing the rationale for clinical work with families.

This approach, although formal and academic in its overall ambience, continued Cohen's thematic emphasis on direct experience. While Terkelsen was delivering a critique of the old paradigm, he was also revealing his own part in the unwinding of that orientation. He was careful not to deride the purveyors of those ideas. Rather, he highlighted the intention of the early investigators to find some active, powerful social intervention with which to deal with the horrors of schizophrenia. He was open about his own early adherence to and endorsement of these models and about the difficulties of the transition to the new paradigm. We knew that it was possible that Dr. Solomon or other members of the faculty might still be teaching those models and deliberately represented ourselves not as experts or as critics, but as fellow colleagues struggling as faculty and students struggle to soften the impact of these terrible illnesses and to stimulate or enable the recovery process.

The second part of the academic side of the workshop centered on presentation of concepts of the new paradigm that are relevant to the design of clinical services for families of the long-term mentally ill.

Terkelsen told students that he and others who had become skeptical about Type one models were turning increasingly to family surveys as a point of departure. Reviewing survey literature including Creer and Wing (1974) and Hatfield (1983) and his own experience consulting with families, he told students that families looked for three basic kinds of assistance from professionals: 1) information about the illness and about the methods of treatment, 2) specific advice and guidance in responding to the problems inherent in relating to the mentally ill member, and 3) acknowledgment, support, and respect for the emotional toll of the illness (including the ill person's response to the illness) on the family. He pointed out that although not an exhaustive list, these three requests recurred in all the available surveys. He linked these data to other universes of experience by noting that the same three requests appear in surveys of families fac-

ing crises that are not directly related to mental illness, such as natural disasters, physical illness, and death. He concluded that in the
absence of other solid empirical foundations, the strategy of asking
families what they would like to receive has produced a convergence
of opinion from which it is possible to derive a rationale for family
services that come closer to meeting the needs of families than do
old-paradigm interventions.

This part of the presentation was very much for the benefit of
the faculty. We assumed that some members of the faculty might
persevere in the old paradigm regardless of its impact on families.
But Terkelsen was charting the course through the transition period
for any faculty who continued to teach the old paradigm more from
lack of a compelling alternative than from any special devotion to the
ideas.

Terkelsen continued by demonstrating in detail how a professional
can give information about schizophrenia, information that is readily
understandable to lay persons and that goes a long way toward taking the mystery out of the illness. First, he identified negative symptoms as particularly problematic for families to live with and
understand and developed a model of withdrawal and amotivational
states founded on the psychophysiology of stimulus barrier functions.
He recalled descriptions of these states in Cohen's personal account
and explained the use of psychopharmacological interventions in
light of this model. Then he reviewed the longitudinal outcome studies, highlighting how these studies had altered the prevailing professional view about the long-term prognosis and about the importance
of long-term community-based psychosocial services.

All of this was done as a demonstration of how professionals can
talk to families about schizophrenia. The language was deliberately
nontechnical. There was ample use of visuals and handouts to enhance
concept formation. Reference was made repeatedly to the role of social
workers, specifically Anderson and Hogarty (Anderson et al. 1986),
in the development of this kind of educational experience for families.
It was at the same time a short course on the biological basis of schizophrenia for students and faculty, in which implications were apparent
both for work with families and for the design of psychosocial programming for schizophrenic patients. The academic side of the workshop supplied immediate answers to the students' need to know what
they could do and pointed optimistically toward a distinctive role for
social work in the care of the chronically mentally ill. This latter aspect
was especially important in our efforts to make contact with the institution, because the faculty were mainly interested in the implications
of the team's presentation for a course on the practice of social work.

Plenty of time was left at the end of the workshop for questions
and discussion. Throughout this part of the workshop, we worked

together, linking some academic point with a part of the personal account. This type of interchange had the effect of weaving the two parts of the workshop into a whole. Additionally, it gave the students and faculty an opportunity to witness a relative and a clinician collaborating in a condition of mutual respect. We each acceded to the experiential base of the other. And in doing so, we each confirmed the authority of the other as a teacher to the students and to the faculty.

THE STUDENTS RESPOND

Students were very interested in the accounts of favorable long-term outcomes. One young man described how depressing it had been for him to be assigned to work with the chronically mentally ill without this kind of perspective. One young woman exclaimed, "I wish my parents could be here to hear you," and then, with a great deal of emotion, shared with her classmates that her sister had been mentally ill for many years. These responses served to further authenticate the team's message in the eyes of the faculty.

THE FACULTY RESPONDS: AN INVITATION FOR RETURN ENGAGEMENTS

Immediately on completion of the workshop, Dr. Solomon asked if we could return to give the workshop in the other second-year practice classes. She contemplated six return engagements and felt that the experience would be extremely useful for the other students. This entailed a change in strategy, because the original intent of the committee was to go from one school to another, and it was immediately apparent that this one school would consume all the available energies of the team for that academic year. After a brief caucus, we agreed to return, noting that something very favorable was in the air at Columbia and estimating that this was perhaps the most effective way to rapidly make substantive contact with a majority of the faculty. In subsequent classes, we followed the same basic format. Cohen found, however, that it was tremendously wearing to retell a personal story again and again and therefore evolved a collage of anecdotes, some from her own experience and others she knew from support group meetings of her local AMI chapter. In subsequent presentations, Terkelsen deemphasized the critique of the old paradigm and expanded on the explication of ideas from the new paradigm.

In each instance, it appeared that the visits of the team had been picked up in the informal faculty and student grapevines so that positive anticipations around the workshop built with each repetition. In several other classes, students revealed direct experience with mental illness in a family member, again conveying a sense that we had fostered a benevolent ambience in the classrooms. Additionally, the faculty had rearranged their teaching schedules to include the workshop while the other course work on mental illness was still alive in the students' experience. This step, together with active faculty participation and open endorsement of the team's message, suggested to the students that our presentation was an integral part of the school's curriculum.

COMMUNICATING OUR INTEREST IN PROMOTING INSTITUTIONAL CHANGE

Through this series of classroom visits, the team had made contact with the majority of the second-year faculty of one school of social work. Yet our aim was to promote incorporation of new-paradigm perspectives and experiences into the culture of the institution. Knowing that we had made a very solid beginning on the road toward that end, we met with Dr. Solomon—over lunch, between classes—and raised the larger agenda and obtained her commitment to a follow-up process. At an evaluation and planning meeting in the spring of 1985 with Dr. Solomon and Dean Gitterman, we found a warm reception and two enthusiastic advocates. Indicating their delight with the workshop as a learning experience ("You were a breath of fresh air"), they invited the team to return for the same cycle the following year. We reminded them that the original intent of the involvement with Columbia was to promote institutional acceptance of fresh and more enabling approaches to families and to the mentally ill and confirmed the committee's desire to provide AMI teams to the school until teaching in this content area was a part of the school's curriculum. Dean Gitterman suggested that the team give thought to videotaping a presentation for classroom use. We indicated that it was more than likely that additional people could be recruited for the Columbia project from the membership of local AMI affiliates and that we preferred this more personal approach. Dean Gitterman offered to make introductions to key faculty at other schools of social work, saying, "You don't have to go and sell yourselves. I can do the calling." Finally, we were asked to comment on the school's basic reading list in the area of the family and mental illness.

INVOLVING THE SCHOOL IN THE ALLIANCE: A JOINT WORKSHOP

Meanwhile, it was apparent to us that much more personpower would be required to do the work of the committee. Encouraged by the first-year experience at Columbia and anticipating an invitation to return, Cohen made arrangements for the committee to give the workshop "Promoting Attitudinal Change in Professional Schools" at the annual conference of AMI of New York. The intent was to take this opportunity to recruit AMI members for participation in the Columbia project. In anticipation of that task, Terkelsen invited Dr. Solomon to present the school's experience at the workshop. The intent was twofold. First, this was an opportunity to demonstrate for the membership of AMI an instance of positive collaboration between one school and one AMI team. Second, the team believed that Dr. Solomon's participation in such an event, including exposure to other members of AMI and to other and more vigorous opinions about the importance of curricular change in the professional schools, would deepen her interest in permanent curricular change within her own school. The scale of the annual conference, together with the intensity of adverse opinion about professionals expressed, took her by surprise and may have contributed to her sense of importance of the project.

By the beginning of November of 1985, the pool of AMI members who were ready to participate in the second cycle of the Columbia project far exceeded the number needed for a full complement. Additionally and to our surprise, three professionals who had attended the AMI of New York workshop volunteered to participate for the academic side of the presentations.

At about this time, two other schools of social work in the New York area approached the committee with requests for speakers. At least one of these requests grew out of Dean Gitterman's voluntary efforts to advertise the work of the committee among his colleagues at other schools. Thus, by the time we were ready to begin the second Columbia cycle, it was clear that the committee's team approach to promoting institutional change was alive and well, both in terms of available AMI personpower and in terms of requests for visits to the schools.

ASSESSMENT OF THE SECOND COLUMBIA CYCLE

In the second cycle, we again went into seven classes, involving seven AMI members and two outside professionals. In a follow-up assessment meeting, most of the participants agreed that this had been a very strong, emotionally charged experience. Some had found the experience particularly draining and questioned, "Do you have to parade all your agony?" Those who found the experience easier, even supportive, reported that they had shared selectively and prepared their presentation beforehand, even to the point of rehearsing with other family members. All agreed that the warm reception and support on the part of the faculty made for a positive experience.

At this writing, in conjunction with word spreading about the Columbia experience or through other channels, three other schools of social work in the New York area have initiated requests for visits by AMI teams. Some will present to student classes. Some will present to the entire student and faculty body in special conferences. Others will present exclusively to the faculty. As we move into this expanded phase of the New York project, several issues will have to be addressed. First, how are we to select AMI volunteers? Although some people are presumably more inherently skillful at this kind of advocacy than others, the open democratic and participative nature of AMI makes it difficult to select some over others. More frequent and more extensive training sessions might lead to more appropriate forms of voluntarism.

Second, we are still at the beginning of the realization of our long-range goal of impacting in a lasting way on the curriculum and on the culture of the schools we are visiting. At Columbia, we have agreed to return for a third cycle and yet are attempting to respond to requests from three other schools with limited personpower. Clearly, we do not have the resources to mount the kind of efforts at the other schools that we have done and can do at Columbia.

Third, we have heard from students that, in their fieldwork assignments, students are often confronted with a very different point of view from the one they are getting in our workshops. Here we are up against the limitations of a local effort in effecting change at a level beyond that of a single institution. We like to think of the efforts of the Curriculum and Training Committee as interdigitating with efforts of the Public Awareness Committee and other elements of AMI that impact more broadly on attitudes toward families of the mentally ill.

REFERENCES

Anderson CM, Reiss DJ, Hogarty GE: Schizophrenia and the Family: a Practitioner's Guide to Psychoeducation and Management. New York, Guilford, 1986

Creer C, Wing JK: Schizophrenia at Home. London, Institute of Psychiatry, 1974

Hatfield AB: What families want of family therapists, in Family Therapy in Schizophrenia. Edited by McFarlane WR. New York, Guilford, 1983, pp 41–65

Commentary to Chapter 7

Teaching Psychiatrists About the Family's Experience

Christian C. Beels, M.D.

Cohen and Terkelsen present with moving restraint an adventure into unknown territory: entering a professional school with a personal as well as a scientific message from the consumers. In some ways, a school of social work may be less of a moated castle than, say, a psychiatric residency program—social workers are, after all, supposed to start where the client is and are more prepared than members of most disciplines to think of the family as the client. Nevertheless, the authors discovered, and describe very well, the tension generated by crossing boundaries and presenting a new paradigm in a strange place. From my own experience, I recognized especially the moment when people in the class identify themselves as relatives who have faced the same ordeal, so that from that point on, the we-they, trainer-trainee, and provider-consumer roles are all mutable, and an extraordinary recognition of common humanity takes place.

Beyond that first encounter, it seems to me that the strategy presented of gradually introducing the two organizations to each other is clearly effective—a model of tact and careful building of confidences. What I have to add in this commentary is not at all a criticism of what Cohen and Terkelsen present, but rather an expansion of it. I will also raise some questions about what will happen in other contexts and perhaps later on in schools of social work after the new paradigm has moved a little further into history and is not so new.

What I have to say is based on 10 years teaching the family's experience (through observed interviews with family members and through the direct supervision of multiple-family groups) in a community service that is part of a psychiatric residency training program.

217

I have also had 5 years of teaching a variety of psychoeducational approaches to Fellows in Public Psychiatry—young psychiatrists who will go out and run the public clinics where most contact with chronic patients and their families takes place. And of course, I have learned a great deal from the observation of my colleague William McFarlane's carefully constructed program for the training of on-line professionals in state and county aftercare clinics all over New York (in press). His approach is based on Carol Anderson's workshop and single-family design (Anderson et al. 1986), plus his own experience with multiple-family groups.

This experience tells us that it is possible to teach the new paradigm of working with the family, from the top, so to speak, rather than introducing it from the outside, if the members of the faculty responsible for teaching about schizophrenia have been reading the literature and have a commitment to altering practice accordingly. We have been teaching this point of view in the Columbia residency program at the Psychiatric Institute since I arrived in 1975 to assume the position of Director of Training on the Community Service. Dr. Terkelsen and several others joined me on that service, and we have trained a lot of residents in combining educational and family work. I have some evidence that the social work students and psychology interns who passed through are also applying this profamily philosophy in the clinics and hospitals in which they work.

Let me briefly list here, for comparison with Cohen and Terkelsen's experience, some of the tactics that were available to us as designers of training. 1) A biweekly clinical conference on the inpatient unit where a family was interviewed was instituted. The residents were put on notice that this had nothing to do with the teaching of family dynamics or conventional family therapy. The purpose was to get the family to teach us what they had been through in coping with the illness, what information they needed from us to cope further, and what institutional support we could plan with them for the future. There was as much respectful on-the-spot psychoeducation built into this interview as possible. 2) Residents were required to colead a multifamily group in the outpatient department, under the supervision of an experienced nonmedical staff person who was the group's continuing therapist and consultant. This gave them a firsthand experience of family coping, of what advice was helpful and what was not, and especially of the long time frame in which therapeutic activists must learn to think about the changes in the lives of patients and families. 3) I did an exercise with each new group of trainees in which I asked them to recall a time when a member of a group they had been in (e.g., camp, college, retreat) had become psychotic. One person out of 10 has always had this experience and is willing to talk about it. Reviewing the experience of the group—the demoralization and, at the same time, the intense feeling of responsibility—makes it clear that families are not the only human group that has these responses to psychosis in a member. 4) The trainees had as strong a dose of reading and discussion of the current literature as class time would permit.

As these efforts were building up over the years, I began to see that there is an important difference between being on the outside, trying to bring the news to perhaps insensitive or hardened insiders, and being on the inside. As my point of view became recognized, I had the responsibility of addressing these problems in the open marketplace of ideas that is the curriculum of the residency training program or the postresidency fellowship. In this later stage, things become more complicated than they are when the purpose is to direct the trainees' attention to something they had not thought about before.

It will not do, for example, to be simply anti-deinstitutionalization or anti–family therapy. Both are here to stay, and both are very complex, as a look at the works of Bachrach (1983) and Anderson et al. (1986), to name only two, will show. If you are in the professional training business, you have to keep looking to the literature for complications and contradictions. Let me give some examples here of the kinds of things that we need to think about.

There are some patients who do not respond to medication and social support, or indeed to medication and straightforward family support. Hospitalization does not help much either, and anyway they are quickly released from hospitals as hospitals are now organized. Who are these families and patients who frustrate our most enlightened and profamily approaches, who won't come to our multifamily groups, or who prefer street drugs or no drugs to ours? These patients for whom our standard programs do not work are a small part of the total, but they may use up a majority of the service's time, energy, and budget. Certainly they are the patients that residents and fellows most urgently present at case conferences.

Clearly, these patients are not all the same: our failures testify even more clearly than our successes to the wide variety of clinical pictures that still come under the description of schizophrenia. In this great variety, three very different and instructive kinds of failures stand out from my experience of running case conferences.

One is a kind of renegade, wandering, revolving-door patient, whom Pepper and Ryglewicz (1984) and others have called the young adult chronic patient. Whatever this unhappy and tempestuous person's connection with family may be—painfully close or alienated—there is in the history a lack of socialization into a patient role, either in a hospital or an outpatient program. Bachrach (1984) has pointed out the double message we give these young people: we tell them to stay out of the hospital to avoid being stigmatized as a patient, but on the other hand, we have no other community or role to offer them. To this environmental anomie the patients add a rebelliousness of their own, perhaps part youth and part temperament, and the result is systematic defeat of whatever we have to offer, even if, later in their career, we offer something very good. There seems to be an early program-personality interaction here that is fateful for the course and has nothing to do with family or medication. Test has begun to investigate what social measures it takes to work successfully with very difficult people like this, including those with a history of substance abuse (Test et al. 1989).

A second kind of instructive failure appears when in addition to schizophrenia there is both a characterologic problem in the patient and an overinvolvement on the part of the family such that all our efforts to offer straightforward education, rehabilitation, and medication are frustrated. The more constructive support we provide, the worse things get. In these cases, we really have learned something from the strategic and systemic family therapists about how to proceed. This does not mean that the family caused the problem in the first place, but it does mean that loosening the family's grip on the solution makes progress possible.

The most instructive failure of all of course is that which arises from misdiagnosis. Anyone who has made an academic career from teaching the management of schizophrenia has seen the definition of that word shrink, dissolve, split, and practically vanish as other entities are differentiated from it. Often, as in the case of bipolar affective disorder, this has been accompanied by a successful drug treatment of the disorder that is split off. So we have to be very careful of becoming dogmatic in our definition of schizophrenia and in our certainty that we have a simple model of it to present to our students and our patients and their families. Discoveries next year could prove us wrong, or at least wrong about a large fraction of what we thought were a homogeneous group of patients.

This is just as true of social-environment investigation as it is of biological-pharmacological investigation. The work of Goldstein (1987) and of Harding et al. (1987) shows that we will learn much about the illness from studying our patients' environments both before the illness began and long afterward. We need to press ahead with research on all fronts—the brain, the microenvironment of the family or the network or the neighborhood, or the institutional macroenvironment. It is clear that we will continue to learn useful things in all these areas. A prejudice against family or social research such as the National AMI and New York AMI have sometimes expressed, although understandable in light of past caricatures of the "schizophrenogenic family," is, in the present climate of research in this field, very destructive of the ends that all of us, families and providers alike, are seeking. Over the long haul, the largest variability in the course of schizophrenia has been found in social factors: not just family factors such as high or low expressed emotion, but program factors such as social support, the availability of partial hospitalization, outreach, and so on. But there is so much we do not know about the way these factors operate that to suspend investigation of them will abort the development of program elements really helpful to patients and families.

I have tried in the above comments to describe the training of professionals in the good news that is coming out about the treatment of schizophrenia, from the vantage point of what I hope is a moderately up-to-date department of psychiatry. My colleagues in that department, especially my boss, the director of Residency Training, would be interested to hear me characterize it so positively, because from the inside I am very critical indeed. But when I visit abroad, I realize we are not so badly off. Certainly we take seriously our obligation to bring the trainees the latest thinking about effective treatment. That effort is very much part of our research orientation. We also try to make contributions to treatment research, and we try to take into account as wide a variety of theories in devising that research as we can. Consequently, we present our trainees with many contradictions, and I know that in their efforts to deal with difficult cases they often do not thank us for it. But we are always trying to make the point that the contradictions between biological, psychological, and social approaches are not really contradictions at all; they add to each other, and to bring them all together is the true job of the clinician.

REFERENCES

Anderson CM, Reiss DJ, Hogarty GE: Schizophrenia in the Family: A Practitioner's Guide to Psychoeducation and Management. New York, Guilford, 1986

Bachrach LL (ed): Deinstitutionalization (New Directions for Mental Health Services No 17). San Francisco, CA, Jossey-Bass, 1983

Bachrach LL: The concept of young adult chronic psychiatric patients: questions from a research perspective. Hosp Community Psychiatry 35:573–580, 1984

Goldstein MJ: The UCLA High-Risk Project. Schizophr Bull 13:505–514, 1987

Harding CM, Brooks GW, Ashikaga T, et al: The Vermont Longitudinal Study of persons with severe mental illness, I: methodology, study sample, and overall status 32 years later. Am J Psychiatry 144:718–735, 1987

McFarlane WR: Multiple family groups and the treatment of schizophrenia, in Handbook of Schizophrenia. Edited by Nasrallah HA. Amsterdam, Elsevier (in press)

Pepper B, Ryglewicz H (eds): Advances in Treating the Young Adult Chronic Patient (New Directions in Mental Health Services No 21). San Francisco, CA, Jossey-Bass, 1984

Test MA, Wallisch LS, Allness DJ, et al: Substance abuse in young adults with schizophrenic disorders. Schizophr Bull 15:465–476, 1989

Chapter 8

A Curriculum Guide for Fieldwork in Chronic Mental Illness

Mona Wasow, A.C.S.W.

Although schools of social work have always had field practicums in mental health, they have not had them specifically in the area of chronic mental illness. The problems in our country for the chronically mentally ill, their families, and society as a whole are now very great. It is important that professionals in all the helping professions be well trained in this area. This chapter describes a curriculum guide used at the University of Wisconsin-Madison School of Social Work, but with minor shifts in emphasis and content, it could be used for the training of other health care professionals as well.

Fieldwork, or practicum, is designed to give social work students practical experience. Students work from 16 to 20 hours a week with the chronically mentally ill and their families and the many agencies and institutions with which they are connected. At the same time, the students take classes at the university, and the overall plan is to link theory to practice and end up with a knowledgeable, skillful practitioner. Students working with chronically mentally ill patients take, among other classes, concurrent courses in psychopathology and methods of social work practice. Students who are working with the aged mentally ill take the above-mentioned courses plus a course in aging and mental health.

The 16–20 hours of fieldwork are supervised by university field faculty and by trained agency social workers. The amount of direct supervision and the amount of autonomy a student has depends on

223

several things: 1) the maturity and abilities of the student, 2) the demands of a particular placement, and 3) the preferred style of supervision by the social workers and faculty instructors involved. Students, agency personnel, and university faculty all stay in close, ongoing contact.

This chapter will describe the content, goals, methods of instruction, and student placements in our fieldwork with the chronically mentally ill. Student development over the year is described, from both instructor and student perspectives, and a picture of what students should know and be able to do by the end of the year is given.

EDUCATIONAL OBSTACLES

Practice often lags many years behind new theoretical developments. In the area of chronic mental illness, this is precisely what we find. Perhaps because they are more attractive for students to study and learn, the psychodynamic models of treating chronically mentally ill patients still have a firm hold in some schools of social work. Another reason for this phenomenon is that many older professors were taught the psychodynamic models so popular in the United States from the 1940s through the mid-1960s. Some professors continue to teach what they were taught because they have not kept abreast of new findings. Consequently, despite the mounting evidence of genetic and biochemical involvement in the etiology of mental illness, there are few schools of social work teaching with this newer knowledge base in mind. The harm this knowledge lag is causing the mentally ill, their families, and society has been documented elsewhere (Hatfield 1979; Lefley 1985; Torrey 1988; Wasow 1982; Wing 1978).

Gerhart (1985), from Rutgers University, made the excellent point that the ultimate goal of most students entering social work is to become psychotherapists with a private practice of their own. I have made this same observation in 18 years of teaching. Social work educators need to redouble their efforts to socialize students to the profession's values and practices of working with the poor and disenfranchised; chronically mentally ill persons are among the most downtrodden in our society. Gerhart (1985) has pointed out that students "readily pick up our overt as well as covert values" (p. 18). "Social work schools . . . have neglected direct practice with the chronically mentally ill . . . in spite of the fact that this group is a large, highly visible, and significant constituency of clients in great need of professional interventions, a constituency in the classical model of social work's concern" (p. 21).

Both Gerhart and I work closely with field agencies. We share with field personnel our academic expertise, and the field-workers share with us and the students their practice expertise. "This seems to me to be the very essence of school and field working together to benefit clients and students" (Gerhart 1985, p. 17).

Atwood (1982) wrote about professional prejudices against the chronically mentally ill: "Mental health clinicians, like the public, are ambivalent toward the mentally ill. Cultural biases contribute to the negative side of this ambivalence, while the ethic of professional service enhances this positive side" (p. 172). Atwood feels we can reduce this prejudice and help stimulate professional pride in treating chronically mentally ill patients.

Student Attitudes

In a review of the research literature on the chronically mentally ill, Rubin (1984) found that students listed these patients as the least appealing of all client groups to work with: "Out of 16 client groups that we asked students about the one which they found least appealing was the chronically mentally ill disabled" (p. 20). Rapp (1985) also made the point that social work students do not want to work with chronically mentally ill patients, but rather want to learn to do insight psychotherapy, "which is not effective with this population and may be toxic." Rapp (1985) stressed that students need to be familiar with DSM-III-R (American Psychiatric Association 1987) and with medications in order to work with chronically mentally ill patients. "Social work has prided itself on its concern on the 'total person,' which has meant its focus on individual, social, and environmental issues. Missing from this formulation has been the attention to the biological and physical" (Rapp 1985, p. 9). This does not mean they have to have a physician's knowledge about medications, but rather that they must know about their importance in treatment, side effects, and compliance issues. Chronically mentally ill patients and their reliance on medications forces us to confront these dimensions. Dincin (1985) made a similar point: "So social workers need to understand about dopamine and serotonin and norepinephrine, and what their reactions and interactions are . . . They need to have a very deep understanding of the side effects of medications and how to handle them" (p. 9). He asked, "What are the implications for social work education in this rather complete revolution in thinking in just one generation of social work education?" (p. 9). His answer was that we need to know brain physiology and its relationship to psychology.

Rapp (1985) feels that as far as the education of our students is concerned, there is no group that raises critical social work issues as clearly as the chronically mentally ill. These issues include:

1. The importance of outreach
2. Families and their needs
3. Environmental interventions and issues
4. Understanding that client changes are gradual and incremental and suffer frequent setbacks
5. The need to see and feel things from the client's perspective
6. Legal and political issues
7. The need for long-term services and a continuum of care
8. The "powerlessness, discrimination, and the difficulty of gaining neighborhood acceptance of our clients" (Rapp 1985, p. 13)

AGENCY BENEFITS

Rapp (1985) and I (1982) have written about how agencies working with the chronically mentally ill have benefited from having students and, consequently, so have the clients they serve. Agencies have been able to provide many hours of service that would not have been possible without student help. In Madison, Wisconsin, our field students who study chronic mental illness have been sought after eagerly in both traditional and nontraditional agencies: in the jail, the shelter for the homeless, special living arrangements, clubs for the chronically mentally ill, group homes, hospitals, day-care centers, and nursing homes for the mentally ill elderly.

Rapp (1985) wrote that the demand for professionals to work with the chronically mentally ill exists and will expand rapidly in the future: "The research on the chronically mentally ill combined with the research in social work practice suggests that we know what to do and what to teach" (p. 46). What is more, we are beginning to know what *not* to teach, e.g., psychodynamic theories about chronic mental illness. He points out curriculum obstacles to teaching well in this area:

1. A lack of faculty with the background and interest to teach about chronic mental illness. Social work educators are now trying to overcome part of this problem through the development and collection of curriculum materials.
2. A lack of good field placements in the area. These surely could be developed, as there is desperate need in the community for care of the chronically mentally ill.
3. A lack of student interest in the area. As mentioned elsewhere, if our professors were truly interested and knowledgeable, the students would follow suit.
4. Most schools of social work prohibit undergraduate programs from specializing; they must be more general. Rapp (1985) sug-

gested that "a course devoted to the chronically mentally ill should not replace existing 'base' courses but is recommended as an addition which some programs can afford" (p. 47).

Dincin (1985), in discussing why we should train students to work with the chronically mentally ill, asked, "Is the field of social work willing to deal once again with the basics of life for a marginally adjusted group, or are we only willing to deal with the intrapsychic issues of the walking well?" (p. 28). There may not be much literature about the need for educating social workers in the field to work with chronically mentally ill patients, but what there is is remarkably consistent in what it sees as important, which leads me to believe we are on the right track.

FIELD PRACTICUM CURRICULUM

Goals

Many social work students enter school with visions of doing insight-oriented psychotherapy with relatively well people. One main goal of our curriculum is to guide students toward seeing the value and status involved in doing the front-line work with those who are in desperate need. Our field environment is not an attractive office in a clinic, with pretty paintings on the wall, and our clientele are not highly motivated, polite people who are grateful for our concern. We work in depressing environments, in run-down rooms and dingy shelters for the homeless, and with people who do not get cured, who sometimes get worse, and who may try to avoid us.

The challenge is to get students to see the value in this work, to admire the chronically mentally ill for their survival skills despite such devastating illnesses and a culture that is prejudiced against them. The challenge is also to get students to honor themselves for wanting to do the work. "Consider the chronic patient: If you had his limitations and handicaps, are you sure you would do as well? So respect the 'crock,' and, as therapist, respect yourself for being of service to him or her" (Loeb 1983, p. 32). A first goal, then, is the process of humanizing chronically mentally ill people, so that we never lose sight of the individuals within the illness. A second goal is to value and upgrade the technology of caring (Loeb 1983), as opposed to thinking in terms of "cure." Students sometimes feel disillusioned and discouraged when they learn that cure is not possible. It is important to value and understand the notion of care from the beginning. It is more heady for a novice to presume to be a magical, curative therapist, but students can derive gratification and satisfaction from caring roles, if they understand why and how important they are.

These are basic humanistic goals underlying all that we do. The next big job is to develop the contents of a curriculum. To be humane, loving, and well intentioned is not enough. To be helpful, professionals need a great deal of knowledge. An outline of the main content areas we study follows.

I. The major mental illnesses, as defined by DSM-III-R (see Kane 1982 for the underlying rationale)
II. Different treatment modalities
    A. Medications
    B. Psychosocial supports—models of community supports
    C. Crisis interventions
    D. Other
III. Community resources—what already exists and what needs to be developed
IV. The deinstitutionalization movement—pros and cons
    A. The history of treating mental illnesses
        1. In the United States
        2. Cross-cultural perspectives
        3. Legal issues, especially commitment laws
V. Different perspectives on mental illnesses
    A. Patient
    B. Family
    C. Societal views in the United States
    D. Cross-cultural
VI. Basic clinical skills
    A. Interviewing clients and families, both individually and in groups
    B. Being able to work with other health care providers and helping systems
    C. Doing a psychosocial assessment
    D. Planning interventions and treatments
    E. Advocacy for clients and their families
    F. Understanding, influencing, and developing policy issues
VII. Keeping abreast of current research

Methods of Instruction

The methods used to achieve these goals are varied and fall into four main categories: 1) the weekly seminar, 2) direct practice in the field, 3) readings and writings, and 4) assignments, both academic and experiential. The average field unit includes 10–15 students.

The weekly seminars run 2½–3 hours every week from September to May. The seminars are used to discuss field concerns, to brainstorm, and to problem solve. The seminar plus a "methods of social work practice" course are our main vehicles for linking theory to practice. Each student is responsible for planning and running one seminar. This is an opportunity for them to go into depth on a topic of their choosing. There is a huge area of topics from which to choose, as long as it has to do with the chronically mentally ill. We have had seminars on stigma, legal issues, medications, drug abuse, family issues, aging, housing problems, sexuality, and many other issues. Needless to say, students do best when they are covering a topic they are particularly interested in.

The student is totally responsible for everything: topic, methods of presentation, calling the seminar to order, keeping track of time, and soliciting feedback at the end. This is a time-consuming responsibility, and one that tends to evoke anxiety in most students. It is also the assignment they complain most about, and praise as the most helpful learning experience . . . after it is over!

Every student has to tell me about his or her topic and plan of instruction 2 weeks before the presentation. I am available to assist them as little or as much as they desire. Some people want very little help. They know exactly what they want to cover and how they plan to do it, and they consult with me for just 15 minutes. Other students want to go through every detail, and we may work together for hours. Either approach, or anything in-between, is fine; students vary a great deal in how they work best, but going over their plans with them first helps ward off poor presentations. It is terribly important for the growth and sense of professional accomplishment of students that they do well in this assignment. It is equally important for the group as a whole, so that they get a lot out of the seminar.

A great deal of attention is paid to the content of the presentation and to teaching techniques. Professionals spend a lot of time teaching, trying to get ideas and information across to clients, colleagues, and the community. For this reason, an emphasis is placed on how best to get content and ideas across. A large variety of teaching techniques are tried out, including lectures, small-group work, guest speakers, clients speaking to us, field trips, our field unit doing presentations in the community, working on advocacy projects (i.e., writing letters to politicians for funding, training volunteers to work with chronically mentally ill patients, working shifts in a shelter for the homeless), and a combination of experiential and academic exercises.

How the seminar hours are divided varies from week to week, depending on both leader and group wishes. A typical seminar is spent as follows: 15 minutes to an hour is given to field issues that may need immediate attention. This always has top priority. It is also a time for general announcements about meetings going on, articles just read, or a special project being developed. Sometimes there is a need to spend time just checking in, complaining about school pressures, asking for reassurance that they really are in the right profession, or telling a good joke. We always aim toward developing a dynamic, safe, warm, strong, and cohesive group. The group is our laboratory for risk taking, sharing, comfort, and intensive learning.

After this first period, the presentation of the week proceeds, with a 10-minute coffee break at the halfway mark. The last 15 minutes are spent giving the presenter feedback. Students tend to be very gentle and supportive of one another. They usually need to be urged to be more critical, but are always told that this is to be constructive criticism. On the few occasions when a presentation is poorly done, the student is given the opportunity to do another one later in the semester. Also, every week a different person brings in refreshments, lending an important element of pleasure and comfort to our unit meetings.

Direct Practice in the Field

The 16–20 hours a week spent working directly with clients, their families, and the mental health system are the "nuts and bolts" of the curriculum. This is where students do most of their learning. There is a large variety of field placements from which to choose, and an effort is made to match students' interests and needs with available placements. A partial list of placements follows:

1. Sheltered workshop for the chronically mentally ill
2. Group homes
3. State and county hospitals
4. The YWCA and YMCA
5. Shelter for the Homeless
6. Jail
7. Special living arrangements for chronically mentally ill patients
8. Model community treatment programs
9. Adult day centers (for chronically mentally ill elderly)
10. A drop-in center (club) for chronically mentally ill patients

Placements vary from highly structured, as in the group homes or hospitals, to unstructured, as in the shelter for the homeless.

Because many of the placements coordinate their efforts, and clients are often involved with more than one agency, students quickly learn about the local mental health system and community resources and how best to use them on their clients' behalf. An effort is made to involve students in as large a variety of activities and experiences as possible. In the course of the year, they have contact with chronically mentally ill patients as individuals and as part of groups and their families. They lead groups for chronically mentally ill patients that cover different topics, such as medications, grooming skills, shopping, cooking, and sexuality, and sometimes students are involved in support groups for families.

Working with existing community resources and developing new resources are important components of the field experience. The Shelter for the Homeless was one recently developed resource that came out of the combined efforts of social work students, local churches, and volunteers. One student developed something new during her first week of fieldwork, where she was working in the craft room of the YMCA with residents, making collages out of seeds. A resident said to her, "We should be eating these seeds, not pasting them. I'm hungry." The student quickly learned more about social security payments, the lack of budgeting and nutritional skills of most chronically mentally ill patients, and their resulting hunger. She then began tapping community resources, looking for free food. She found a tofu store that was willing to donate their leftovers at the end of the week. From there she went to her recipe book, and back to the YMCA to bake tofu cookies with the men, instead of pasting seeds on paper.

One could argue that you do not need a social work degree to bake cookies! But this is an example of a student's ability to think in terms of outreach—connecting people to community resources, nutritional needs, problem solving, and putting them all together in a helpful way—the best of social work practice.

Our students are often the front-line workers in their placements. They are involved in getting the chronically mentally ill who have fallen through the cracks of social services connected to desperately needed services, in developing new, alternative services for the chronically mentally ill, in getting winter coats for those without, in outreach to those terrified behind locked doors, and yes, even in baking nutritious cookies for those who live on potato chips and coffee.

In sensitizing students to the agonies, stresses, and needs of families, an emphasis is placed on reading and on attending meetings of the Alliance for the Mentally Ill (AMI).

Readings and Writings

Books and journal articles are required reading for the first semester to ensure that basic content is covered in the following areas:

1. The chronic mental diseases, especially the schizophrenias, affective disorders, and the dementias

2. Theories of etiology—what is and is not known
3. Various treatment modalities
4. Medications
5. The deinstitutionalization movement—pros and cons
6. Interaction between the mental health and legal systems
7. Chronic mental illness as experienced by the mentally ill (as near as we can imagine it), parental perspectives, and societal perspectives
8. Community resources—the need for a continuum of care

After the first semester of required reading, students can develop their own reading list for the second semester. By the second semester, students have definite ideas about their major area(s) of interest and are encouraged to pursue it. Students learn best what they need and want to know.

Several written assignments are also made. The first is always an analysis of their field placement. This is designed to facilitate learning about their agency; how it works; how it serves clients; where the funding comes from; the values underlying what is being done; the power structure and how they, the students, fit into it; and the various roles people perform.

Students keep daily logs in which they record what they actually do, how they feel in the process, and what they think about it. They are specifically asked to write about their feelings and their cognitive processes. This is designed to link theory to practice and to develop their knowledge base and their professional awareness of themselves and their clients.

Annotated bibliographies are kept on their readings. This helps to focus their learning, keeps me abreast of what they are reading, and, last but not least, helps the instructor develop a good reading list. Annotated bibliographies help the instructor know what books the students find most useful. There are other written assignments that vary from year to year, but the above-mentioned seem most helpful.

Other Assignments

The reading, writing, and seminar assignments have already been mentioned, and of course the hours spent in direct practice are the most essential assignments of all. But there are other assignments that have a significant impact on student learning. These vary from year to year; the variety of assignments that can be made are limitless.

Good assignments have both cognitive and experiential components to them. For example, one week in the field, the assigned topic was stigma. The student in charge invited the entire field unit down to her placement at a club for chronically mentally ill patients. She gave a scholarly 1-hour presentation on the theories of stigma. Then she had us retire to a back room and select clothing to wear from the used clothes room. A few minutes later, we all emerged dressed in the ill-fitting, unmatched shoes and outfits typical of the chronically mentally ill. It felt awful. We were now all given individual assignments, and 2 hours in which to perform them on the streets of our city. I'll never forget mine, because I was emotionally unable to do it. It was to panhandle 35¢ for bus fare. The pain and humiliation of that experience, the stigma, was more than I could handle. I, who had lectured on stigma for years, for the first time had some small idea of what it was really about. Others had similar assignments, e.g., a job interview for a janitorial position, collecting cigarette butts from ashtrays and cans from trash barrels, and standing on the corner talking to oneself. After struggling for 2 hours with our assignments, we returned to the club. There we had a meaningful discussion about stigma. I think none of us will ever forget the experience and will be more sensitive to what the chronically mentally ill must endure at every turn of their lives.

Another example is several students who worked together, very successfully, to develop a citywide bowling league for their clients. Again, the first step was academic: theories about community organization, and how one gets store managers to donate free T-shirts, hot dogs, and bowling alley time. Then the task was to implement theory into practice. It took 7 months, but it worked. The students donated their Sunday mornings to bowl with their clients, which says a great deal about student commitment.

Training volunteers to work with the chronically mentally ill, putting out a calendar with drawings and poetry done by their clients, and putting on a variety show are a few more examples of the many wonderful and creative assignments completed by field students.

Last year's major accomplishments were involvement in running the Shelter for the Homeless (it was the first winter in years that no one froze to death in our streets) and a field unit presentation to AMI. Because this presentation was a powerful experience for the students, let it be told in the words of one who chose to write it up.

"A Night in the Life of a Student"

by Cindy Desch, M.S.S.W.

In March of this year, our field unit spoke to our local Alliance for the Mentally Ill (AMI). Professor Wasow had been asked to speak on the topic of educating students to do social work with the chronically mentally ill. She decided to bring her students rather than talk about them. We had many doubts as we awaited our turn to be the "professional" presenters. It was the first opportunity to speak in front of such a group for many of the students. An hour later it was over, each of us had spoken, and AMI members were coming to the front of the room with compliments and sad stories and in search of an open ear. We had not only taken on the role of professional and had done well, but also had succeeded in breaking through some of the barriers that often exist between mental health professionals and family members. As one AMI member said at the end of our presentation, "If this is an example of the 'New Professionals,' then we indeed have something to be hopeful for."

Field Unit

At the beginning of our field unit, we were not a united group; nor were we enthusiastic about our upcoming work with this population. The reasons each of us had chosen this field unit were varied. Some students have family members who are mentally ill, some were interested in the content area, and others could not get into another unit. We brought with us anxieties, doubts, and concerns about the client population, along with doubts about our own individual abilities. For many, this would be the first time that our social work skills were tested.

The next weeks were the most heart wrenching. We read stories, articles, and studies about the state of the chronically mentally ill, their loneliness, confusion, poverty, and misery. They were becoming people in our minds and hearts. They were no longer people sneered at on the street. Now they had an identity, and our nervous laughter was being replaced by compassion.

At the end of that first semester, we felt more comfortable and competent as professionals. We continued to struggle with the notion of "cure versus care." There is no cure for mental illness, and at times, this became a frustrating reality. There is an enormous need for care in this population. The validity of caring was an issue continually stressed by our field instructor.

AMI Presentation

When the opportunity to speak to the AMI group was presented, many of us had never had the opportunity to speak at a professional meeting. The presentation to AMI would be our proof that we were indeed capable. Our professor had already demonstrated her confidence in our abilities when she asked us to do the speaking ourselves.

One of the potential problems we faced as we walked into that meeting in March was what type of reception we would meet. Over the years, much animosity has existed between families of chronically mentally ill persons and mental health professionals. Some ignorant mental health professionals have believed that mental illness is caused by poor environment, which led to blaming families. Many family members bear the scars of such accusations, and therefore have reason to be angry with professionals.

We spent a number of weeks planning our presentation. Each of us began by choosing a topic that interested us. Topics ranged from working with rural elderly mentally ill to family involvement, value conflicts, drug compliance, stigma, and personal stories. We spoke not as those who had "the" answers on these issues, but rather as those who were aware of the pain of those individuals and their families who were dealing with chronic mental illness. We were genuine, caring, knowledgeable, and enthusiastic about the work that we were doing.

That night an exchange took place: AMI members had given us affirmation and confidence that we had the ability and skills to be good professionals, and we had made clear our commitment to the chronically mentally ill.

Conclusion

The combination of intensive study and direct client contact was invaluable. Field unit seminars provided us with information about theories and research. Fieldwork provided us with the opportunity to experience the human aspects of the knowledge and content we were receiving in seminars. Each of these components is important and teaches skills and content. Combined, they gave the necessary knowledge, experience, and humanity to be effective. That night in March brought the realization of all of these things. We had become competent professionals. Without that opportunity to speak, I believe that many of us would have finished the year lacking extra self-confidence.

STUDENT DEVELOPMENT

Although there is tremendous variation in student abilities and development in the field [There are, of course, some students who are not very good, and some who flunk out. But for the most part, they are caring, competent, and eager to learn.], a few predictable learning patterns do seem to exist. In briefest summary, those patterns are presented in Table 1. To further illustrate the patterns shown in Table 1, excerpts from student logs follow.

Week 1

"For the first time I am to 'rub elbows' with the social outcasts, and I must try to conceal my being uncomfortable. How will I cope with their vacant, staring eyes, behind which lurk immense pain and suffering? I fear for own security when I see them. I feel terribly inadequate."

"How can we teach these people to be independent in a facility structured to encourage dependency? Our purpose is self-defeating—no 'cure,' only maintenance."

"I hope to God I don't flunk out."

Week 7

"I'm learning slowly, that there are some residents I cannot be effective with."

"When I first started working in this area a year ago, I thought a mentally ill person was just a very neurotic person. It took me quite a while to understand the lack of control over stress, the dependencies,

Table 1. Learning patterns in social work students who work with the chronically mentally ill

	Individual students	Field unit	Role of field instructor
Beginning weeks	Tension, doubts, frustrations, fears, self-involvement; plus excitement and eagerness to begin.	Expression of doubts; learning expectations and trying to understand how the systems work. Wanting quick answers. Sharing concerns.	Availability several hours a day. Liaison work with agencies. Emotional support and encouragement. Educational input.
Weeks 5–8	Much reading for content. Broadening their thinking about the chronically mentally ill, societal reactions to them, pros and cons of deinstitutionalization movement, and roles of social work with the chronically mentally ill. Beginning to look at community resources.	Visiting each others' placements; developing group cohesion; lots of moral support, sharing ideas, and enthusiasm.	Educational input. Realistic limit setting. Historical perspectives on chronic mental illness. Increasing student autonomy and responsibility.
End of semester I, 9–15 weeks	Increased knowledge and confidence.	Sharing of ideas, readings, and projects. Much problem solving of field issues. Strong group cohesion and mutual support.	Midyear evaluations with students and agency personnel. Reviewing content. Planning special projects and work assignments for semester II.
Semester II, 4 months	Functioning as autonomous professionals. Active community work; developing special projects. Dedication to the chronically mentally ill and their families.	Continuing development of the above.	Specific projects encouraged. Continued readings and assignments made. Discussions about their future as professionals and how to continue learning on their own. Emphasis on importance of keeping up with research.

and the failure at interpersonal relationships, etc. I had to learn to appreciate small and often temporary changes as being significant."

"When I confessed my fears at the unit meeting, the patience, guidance, and suggestions coming from everyone were so wonderful and helpful! It gave me the courage to go on."

Weeks 10–15
"A mistake I made which caused most of my discomfort when I started the placement was to make assumptions while lacking the proper knowledge about chronic mental illness. I didn't know the philosophy of the deinstitutionalization movement, the problems of the chronically mentally ill, or the practice goals in working with this population."

"It's hard for me now to believe the feelings and thoughts about the chronically mentally ill that I had at the beginning of the semester. Now I enjoy working in my placement and feel my knowledge and practice are important, for a major part of the community treatment movement lies in the hands of social workers."

"I can't believe how much I've learned in just one semester."

A few quotations cannot begin to do justice to all that goes on in the development of students in the second semester. I close this section with a quote from a student at the AMI meeting described by Cindy Desch:

"I admire your sons and daughters so much. When I think of what they are up against: no money, lousy housing, a society that rejects them, and the terrible anxieties that go along with mental illnesses . . . I just marvel at how they go on. And my admiration for you, the parents, has no bounds."

WHAT SHOULD A STUDENT BE ABLE TO DO AFTER A YEAR OF FIELDWORK?

Morris (1977) said, "If social work is courageous enough, it can combine its reform–social action aims with its clinical aims to produce a fully caring system for those who need it" (p. 358). At the end of a year of fieldwork, the student should be competent to

1. Content
   - Identify the major theories used to explain the major chronic mental illnesses: reactive and process schizophrenia, the depressions, and the dementias. Explain these clearly to family members, both what is and is not known.
   - Recognize the effects of chronic mental illness on intellectual, emotional, and functional processes.
   - Know about the major medications used, their pros and cons, and how patients feel about them. Also should be able to con-

duct a good educational session on medications, both for patients and family members.

- Be knowledgeable about treatment modalities, with an emphasis on medications and psychosocial supports in the community.
- Be up-to-date on the latest research findings in all of the above areas, and understand the importance of staying up-to-date throughout their professional careers.
- Be familiar with cross-cultural literature on chronic mental illness.

2. Clinical skills
   - Demonstrate specialized skills for working with chronically mentally ill patients, both individually and in groups.
   - Have a good feel, both cognitively and emotionally, for how people suffering from chronic mental illness may feel; also, for the feelings of family members and some of the current societal views (including cross-cultural).
   - Demonstrate specialized skills for working with other professionals.
   - Perform an accurate psychosocial assessment of a chronically mentally ill person—and know when outside consultation is needed.
   - Have case management skills. Plan effective interventions for treatment and ongoing care.

3. Policy issues
   - Analyze major policy issues and their implications for delivery of services.
   - Understand existing services and programs, and know what still needs to be developed for a given community. Have some idea of how to go about developing such services.
   - Have some community organization skills, especially about funding issues.
   - Understand the need for a continuum of care in the community and a willingness to advocate for it.
   - Have advocacy skills on behalf of the chronically mentally ill and their families.
   - Have knowledge of legal issues.

SUMMARY

It has been my joy and experience to see that the majority of field students in social work do indeed learn the above in the course of a year. Moreover, they combine their learning with compassion and dedication. They come to understand the value of their front-line work and to respect their clients, as well as themselves as professionals.

In the acknowledgments of my book *Coping With Schizophrenia* (Wasow 1982) I wrote, "To my field students in chronic mental illness, who give me the faith that tomorrow will be better." My faith still holds.

REFERENCES

American Psychiatric Association: Diagnostic and Statistical Manual of Mental Disorders, 3rd Edition, Revised. Washington, DC, American Psychiatric Association, 1987

Atwood N: Professional prejudice and the psychotic client. Social Work 27:172–177, 1982

Dincin J: Psychiatric rehabilitation today, in Education for Practice With the Chronically Mentally Ill: What Works? Edited by Bowker JP. Washington, DC, Council of Social Work Education, 1985, pp 18–31

Gerhart UC: Teaching social workers to work with the chronically mentally ill, in Education for Practice With the Chronically Mentally Ill: What Works? Edited by Bowker JP. Washington, DC, Council on Social Work Education, 1985, pp 50–67

Hatfield A: The family as partner in the treatment of mental illness. Hosp Community Psychiatry 30:338–340, 1979

Kane RA: Lessons for social work from the medical model: a viewpoint for practice. Social Work 27:315–321, 1982

Lefley HP: Etiological and prevention views of clinicians with mentally ill relatives. Am J Orthopsychiatry 55:363–370, 1985

Loeb M: On the technology of caring. Unpublished presentation, University of Wisconsin-Madison, April 1983

Morris R: Caring for vs. caring about people. Social Work 25:358, 1977

Rapp CA: Research on the chronically mentally ill: curriculum implications, in Education for Practice With the Chronically Mentally Ill: What Works? Edited by Bowker JP. Washington, DC, Council on Social Work Education, 1985, pp 32–49

Rubin A: Review of the literature on CMI: what works. Paper presented at the Forum on CMI of the Council on Social Work Education, Lawrence, KS, Nov 8, 1984

Torrey EF: Surviving Schizophrenia: A Family Manual, Revised Edition. New York, Harper & Row, 1988

Wasow M: Coping With Schizophrenia. Palo Alto, CA, Science & Behavior Books, 1982

Wing JK: Reasoning About Madness. London, Fakenham & Reading, 1978

Competence-Based Training of Psychiatric Practitioners in the Rehabilitation of the Chronically Mentally Ill

Timothy G. Kuehnel, Ph.D.
Robert Paul Liberman, M.D.

The current shift in treatment and rehabilitation resources by public mental health agencies toward meeting the needs of the chronically mentally ill must be accompanied by innovations in curricula for the education of mental health and rehabilitation trainees and practitioners. Treatment personnel who are channeled into working with the chronic and severely disabling psychiatric disorders will be ineffective at best and will turn cynical and negativistic at worst unless they are first prepared—both attitudinally and technologically—for coping with and helping this challenging population. The fieldwork curriculum for chronic mental illness described by Wasow in the preceding chapter is a constructive step toward providing the knowledge, attitudes, and skills necessary for social work students to find working with the chronically mentally ill a rewarding experience.

In this commentary, we shall place Wasow's fieldwork curriculum in the context of the obstacles that must be overcome in educating mental health and rehabilitation practitioners, the requisite content for curricula, and the importance of "active learning" methods of instruction. Our experience with a curriculum developed and field-tested for psychiatric residents and other mental health professionals, *Psychiatric Rehabilitation of Chronic Mental Patients* (Liberman et al. 1987), will be described, as it is available for widespread dissemination and utilization in preservice, postgraduate, and in-service training.

EDUCATIONAL OBSTACLES

Retarding the development of professionals who are responsive to the needs of the chronically mentally ill and their relatives are the paucity of relevant course work and of interested and knowledgeable instructors in professional training programs for all the mental health and rehabilitation disciplines. Students are not likely to acquire the attitudes and clinical tools appropriate to the needs of the chronically mentally ill in an educational vacuum—they need teachers and mentors to prepare them for the arduous professional tasks of reducing the impairments, disabilities, and handicaps of the over 2 million individuals in the United States with persistent and severe psychiatric disorders. Mental health professionals have generally viewed the treatment of the chronic mental patient as an unrewarding, frustrating experience that offers little hope for positive outcomes (Meyerson 1978).

The broad array of clinical demands placed on treatment and rehabilitation practitioners who work with this multiply handicapped population have increased since deinstitutionalization. The stresses of working with the chronically mentally ill have further escalated as professionals increasingly encounter the new type of young, aggressive, and noncompliant patient (Pepper 1985). The extension of civil rights to the mentally ill through court orders and new commitment laws and fiscal constraints have reduced the duration of hospital treatment and shifted the locus of care to less structured and uncontrolled community settings, where professionals feel unprotected and helpless in orchestrating the multitude of services required by chronically ill patients. At the same time, the specialized training of professionals in this area has been neglected (White and Bennett 1981; Lefley and Cutler 1988).

These difficulties are reflected in a recent survey in Texas of 436 mental health professionals' attitudes toward chronically mentally ill patients (Mirabi et al. 1985). Eighteen percent of the respondents were psychiatrists, 17% were psychologists, 16% were social workers, 14% were caseworkers, 7% were nurses, and the remainder were allied mental health professionals. Eighty-five percent of the respondents endorsed the view that the chronically mentally ill are not a preferred population to treat, and 68% agreed that most clinicians do not receive adequate training in caring for this population. Eighty-three percent agreed that burnout is common when treating this population, and 73% of the respondents felt that patients are too often treated by a

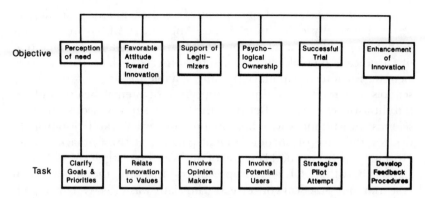

Figure 1. Objectives and tasks required to overcome barriers to adoption of innovation.

sole therapeutic regimen when they need a combination of treatment strategies. Similarly, the Western Interstate Commission on Higher Education found that faculty of graduate education programs rated their interest and competence in working with the chronically mentally ill lower than for any other client group or mental health problem (Moore and Davis 1984). Clearly, the problems that Wasow identified for social workers are shared by all professional disciplines.

An additional educational obstacle is the lag between research and practice, a problem endemic to all mental health disciplines (Glaser et al. 1983). Even in the rational prescription and judicious dosing of psychotropic drugs, new developments in psychopharmacology are adopted slowly and inadequately by psychiatrists (Tupin 1985; Kane 1985). Barriers to the dissemination and adoption of innovative psychosocial interventions for the chronically mentally ill are even greater (Backer et al. 1986; Liberman and Phipps 1987; Kuehnel et al. 1986). Innovative psychosocial interventions are typically complex, demanding, extended in time, and linked to team implementation.

Therefore, factors related to systemwide or organizational changes and innovation adoption should be addressed in the education and training of all mental health disciplines. In addressing these factors, the goal would not be to make the students expert change agents, but rather to acquaint them with those factors that can facilitate or impede the implementation of innovative psychosocial interventions. Figure 1 briefly summarizes the objectives and tasks that need to be addressed to overcome barriers to adoption of innovations. Each of these objectives is based on principles drawn from the planned change literature (Search Institute 1984; Glaser et al. 1983).

Of the various mechanisms for linking innovations to practice, the use of an active learning process in educational programs is of paramount importance. Consequently, researchers and practitioners at the University of California, Los Angeles, (UCLA), working together on problems and solutions for the treatment and rehabilitation of chronically mentally ill patients, have forged a skills-oriented curriculum for interdisciplinary training suitable for use in professional schools and for the continuing education of mental health and rehabilitation clinicians. Because the curriculum was designed by scientist-practitioners who had ongoing experience and responsibilities for the care of chronic mental patients at the Camarillo State Hospital, the Brentwood Division of the West Los Angeles VA Medical Center, and the UCLA Neuropsychiatric Institute, the gap between research and practical concerns of clinicians was effectively bridged.

EDUCATIONAL OBJECTIVES AND CURRICULUM CONTENT

Attaining behavioral skills required for implementing empirically validated treatment modalities for the chronically mentally ill is the overriding goal of the curriculum in *Psychiatric Rehabilitation of Chronic Mental Patients*. As pointed out by Wasow in the preceding chapter, basic humanistic precepts as well as knowledge and familiarity with the needs of the chronically mentally ill help to guide students' values, attitudes, and front-line efforts with this population. However, attitudinal change without being equipped with validated treatment skills will leave students and practitioners handicapped in their clinical work. Treatment research with the chronically mentally ill has shown that it is not how much attention and enthusiasm is offered to patients by staff, but how that attention is structured and given that makes the difference in outcomes (Paul and Lentz 1977).

Thus, after being provided with a conceptual grasp of chronic mental disorders and their rehabilitation using a "stress-vulnerability-coping-competence" model (see Glynn and Liberman, Chapter 9, this volume), trainees are exposed to the specific assessment and treatment skills that have been found effective with the severely psychiatrically disabled. The assessment and treatment skills taught to trainees have as their goals

1. To ameliorate the positive symptoms of a disorder that do not remit with drug treatment
2. To maintain the gains made by the patient during acute treatment and to prevent or delay the reemergence of symptoms over the long haul
3. To assist patients, relatives, and other care givers in managing and reducing the negative or deficit symptoms of major mental

disorders, which pose a largely unanswered challenge to the phar-
macopoeia

4. To inculcate or restore social and living skills that may never have
    been learned or that may have atrophied during periods of illness
    and hospitalization
5. To modify the patient's social environment toward more sup-
    portive and less stressful qualities

Following this rationale, the curriculum provides students with
observable and measurable increases in knowledge and skills in the
following content areas.

**Methods used to conduct diagnostic and symptom-based assess-
ments.** Excerpts from the Present State Examination and the Brief
Psychiatric Rating Scale are used to illustrate the benefits of careful
diagnosis based on operational criteria, standard definitions, and
structured interview formats. The importance of accurate diagnostic
and symptom-based assessment in selecting, timing, and titrating elements of comprehensive treatment for the chronically mentally ill is
also covered.

Methods for functional assessment and planning goals. Functional
assessment assists in the identification of behavioral assets, excesses,
and deficits that help or hinder a patient's performance in social and
occupational roles. Behaviors are identified in terms of frequency,
intensity, duration, latency, form or quality, and timeliness of occur-
rence. Behaviors identified in the functional assessment may be used
to set short- and long-term goals, monitor progress, and determine
optimal rehabilitation outcomes.

**Principles and practical aspects of psychopharmacology appropri-
ate to the needs of the chronically mentally ill.** This area covers
significant points in the judicious use and specific application of psychiatric drugs. An overview is provided on their effects—both desir-
able and undesirable—and practical tips are given on maximizing
compliance while utilizing minimal effective dosages. Guidelines are
offered for use of specific medications to achieve therapeutic effects,
use of drugs to treat side effects, and the importance of individualizing
drug treatment to the patient.

Principles and techniques of social skills training. It is well documented that the chronically mentally ill have difficulty in social functioning. Social skills training is a structured intervention designed
specifically to teach more effective interpersonal behavior. It employs

modeling, role-playing, and in vivo practice, in a manner analogous to teaching a motor skill, such as dancing. In addition to interpersonal behaviors, this structured form of intervention may be used to teach independent living skills in the areas of medication management, leisure and recreation, grooming and personal hygiene, good conversation, symptom self-management, finding and maintaining a home, using public transportation, food preparation, using community agencies, friendship and dating, and job maintenance.

Education of patients and relatives in the nature of chronic mental disorders and training them in communication and problem-solving skills.   Family members and patients are taught about the stress-diathesis model of illness, the course of the disorder, the major symptoms, prodromal symptoms, medication treatment and side effects, and the role of the family in relapse prevention. In addition to didactic psychoeducation, great emphasis is placed on modeling, role-playing, and in vivo practice of new behaviors. These active learning techniques, similar to social skills training, enable the family unit to communicate more effectively about what they like, to request changes in what they do not like, and to effectively solve problems as they occur.

Prevocational and vocational rehabilitation strategies.   Difficulty in obtaining and maintaining employment is a major problem for psychiatric patients. This section emphasizes that work is both an outcome and determinant of the course of chronic mental disorders. Techniques covered include assessment of vocational skills; assessment of and training in prevocational skills such as promptness and getting along with fellow workers and supervisors; training in a specific job, skill, or trade; the use of sheltered employment and transitional employment; finding skills that include soliciting job leads, writing resumes, filling out applications, and interviewing; and maintaining a job. The use of a forum for learning the skills, job searching, and providing social support—the Job Club—is highlighted as a viable technique in this area.

Care and treatment of the chronically mentally ill through a comprehensive system of care.   The 10 necessary services to be provided by an adequate community support program are described. Four of these necessary services are emphasized: 1) Case management is presented as a method to coordinate the range of services needed by the chronically mentally ill. 2) Residential alternatives to provide the least restrictive housing for a patient are described. 3) Crisis intervention with a goal of rapid restabilization of a patient's symptoms and social adjustment are delineated. 4) The psychosocial club model is presented as a method to increase mentally ill persons' (members') levels of effective personal and social contributions on a daily basis.

The content areas of this curriculum reflect the consensus of the field as described in the presentations at the Second National Conference on the Chronic Mental Patient in 1984 (Liberman and Phipps 1987). They also reflect the recommendations of the RSA/National Institute of Mental Health work group for improving vocational services to persons with severe psychiatric disability and the American Psychiatric Association's Task Force on Treatment of Psychiatric Disorders (Liberman et al. 1989).

Based on 15 years of psychiatric practice comprising comprehensive rehabilitation, these seven content areas have been developed into a text, video, and instructor's syllabus that may serve as key resources for delivering the curriculum content to trainees. The text (Liberman et al. 1987) offers practical guidelines and treatment options that can be readily grasped and implemented. These guidelines and treatment options are abundantly illustrated with case examples and learning exercises for the reader. The instructor's syllabus provides a detailed plan and handouts and transparencies for teachers of courses or in-service training. The professionally produced video, awarded First Prize at the International Rehabilitation Film Festival, provides graphic examples of each of the seven areas of practical rehabilitation.

METHODS OF INSTRUCTION

Wasow nicely explicates various innovative instructional techniques that help students link theory to practice via seminar activities, field placements, readings and writings, and cognitive and experiential assignments. To her excellent methods of instruction we would add active-directive teaching methods, which are used to deliver the content and reach the educational objectives of the course outlined in *Psychiatric Rehabilitation of Chronic Mental Patients*.

The active-directive teacher uses learning theory and behavioral training principles to inculcate skills in trainees and students. In turn, the trainees and students are engaged in an active process of learning. Teacher and student together participate in 1) setting precise objectives, 2) brief instruction, 3) modeling with discriminative cuing, 4) behavioral rehearsal with prompting and shaping, 5) performance feedback, and 6) generalization and maintenance of skills. A fuller description of these techniques, with actual examples from the curriculum in *Psychiatric Rehabilitation of Chronic Mental Patients*, is provided in Table 1. A body of research literature supports the effectiveness

Table 1. Description and examples of active-directive teaching components

Component	Description	Example
Setting precise objectives	Three types of objectives may be set: 1) attitudinal, 2) cognitive, and 3) behavioral. All should be behaviorally specific, limited, realistic in terms of time allotted, and appropriate to the knowledge and skill repertoire of participants.	Trainees will score an average of 15 points higher on the "Opinions About Mental Illness Scale" after the completion of the training (attitudinal). Trainees will be able to specify the major benefits of antipsychotics and differentiate acute effects from long-term preventive effects (cognitive). Trainees will demonstrate competent utilization of 8 of 10 therapist skills used in conducting social skills training (behavioral).
Brief instruction	Presentations of didactic material should be brief, highlighted with relevant clinical examples and should follow a general-to-specific hierarchy.	"The three main factors affecting mental disorders are 1) psychobiological vulnerability, 2) socioenvironmental stressors, and 3) protective factors. A clinical example of a socioenvironmental stressor is illustrated by the case of Bob. Bob's first acute episode occurred following the loss of a job . . ."
Modeling with discriminative cuing	Modeling, whether by film or demonstration, should be brief in that only 2–4 "key" competencies should be demonstrated at one time. Discriminative cuing refers to asking the trainees to note or watch for critical therapist behaviors that will occur. The students need to know what they are looking for in	"As you watch the next 4–5 minutes of video, note what the therapist is doing" (otherwise many will be absorbed in following the actions of the patient). Questions may be asked to help the trainees identify and integrate what they observed. For example, "How did the therapist identify a behavioral deficit in

continued

Table 1. Description and examples of active-directive teaching
components *(continued)*

Component	Description	Example
Modeling with discriminative cuing *(continued)*	the demonstration. A competency checklist of key therapist behaviors may be used to "cue" the trainees to the specific behaviors of interest.	need of remediation?" "What question(s) were asked?"
Behavior rehearsal with prompting and shaping (role-playing)	The students/trainees practice the therapist competencies using simulated clinical vignettes. Clear instructions as to roles and specific steps to follow should be given. One or two behaviors at a time should be focused on. The actual rehearsal should be brief. As the instructor, you may need to prompt via gestures or brief verbalization, to help the trainee to initially exhibit the therapist behaviors of interest. Shaping refers to the process of teaching the correct response by encouraging successive approximations to the correct response.	"Today we're going to use behavior rehearsal to practice and learn how to teach patients to make a positive request." The three elements of "making a positive request" are 1) look at the person— make eye contact; 2) say exactly what you would like that person to do; and 3) tell him or her how it would make you feel. Have the trainees form groups of three. Have each group select persons to enact the roles of patient, therapist, and the patient's interpersonal "target." The therapist then would teach the patient how to make a positive request.
Performance feedback	It's important that feedback (from the instructor or other trainees) be positive and behaviorally specific. Rather than negative feedback, suggest alternatives. Usually two or three alternatives are enough (don't overload trainee with feedback).	"I liked the way you specifically asked the patient to tell you what he needs to do differently to help solve the problem he is having with his roommate. Let's try it again and this time have the patient identify the pros and cons of his action after he specifies what he will attempt to do in that situation."

continued

Table 1. Description and examples of active-directive teaching components *(continued)*

Component	Description	Example
Generalization and maintenance of skills	It's not enough for trainees to acquire skills in the classroom. Generalization refers to a student's ability to use these skills in various situations with a variety of patients and problems. Maintenance refers to the continued use of these skills over time. In vivo practice and homework assignments are two ways to promote generalization and maintenance of skills. Homework assignments are likely to be successful if you specify time, place, and materials; promptly take care of potential interfering problems; make your expectations clear; and specify a due date and permanent product.	"Between now and our next class, I'd like you to select one patient from your caseload that you can use these skill-building procedures with. Please complete the first part of the homework completion form now. Select a client who will be amenable to this approach and write his or her name in the blank. Briefly describe the skill you want to teach and specify the methods you're likely to use."

of active-directive training for a wide range of skills with diverse trainee groups (Matarazzo 1978; Kuehnel and Flanagan 1984; Brophy 1986).

Active-directive teaching methods can be flexibly packaged to convey curricula in brief, time-limited workshops or in semester-long seminars. Since 1981, the UCLA faculty of the Clinical Research Center for Schizophrenia and Psychiatric Rehabilitation have delivered the curriculum on chronically mentally ill patients to psychiatric residents as part of their core education at the UCLA Department of Psychiatry and to interdisciplinary audiences at institutions and agencies throughout the United States. The syllabus and video from *Psychiatric Rehabilitation of Chronic Mental Patients* have been used in educational programs ranging from a half-day intensive workshop to a year-long course. The content and amount of active-directive teaching provided can be expanded or contracted to meet the needs and constraints of most professional schools and agencies serving the chronically mentally ill.

Table 2. Pre- versus postworkshop mean scores and standard deviations on measures of knowledge of and attitude toward treatment and rehabilitation of the chronically mentally ill patient

	Preworkshop	Postworkshop	P
General content mastery (knowledge)	22.96 ± 1.9	27.01 ± 2.0	$<.01$
Attitude scale	73.5 ± 18.2	79.9 ± 21.7	$<.05$

Note. Values are means $\pm$ SD.

As an example of this flexible approach to instructional programming, the clinical skills required for training chronically mentally ill patients in social and independent living have been conveyed in a practicum that involves psychiatric residents in an ongoing social skills training group for patients. Meeting weekly for 90 minutes, the group is led by a psychiatrist experienced and skilled in conducting this type of training, thereby offering the residents an experienced role model. A wide variety of patients enter this open-ended group, each being helped to pinpoint skills deficits, set goals, and go through behavior rehearsal, modeling, and reinforcement procedures. After several sessions of observing the experienced leader, the psychiatric residents begin to take on coleadership responsibilities, ultimately becoming autonomous and competent leaders in their own right. This expansion of the skills training component of the curriculum has led trainees into career choices related to clinical and academic work with chronically mentally ill patients (Hierholzer and Liberman 1986).

EVALUATION OF THE CURRICULUM

A 2-day workshop, a version of *Psychiatric Rehabilitation of Chronic Mental Patients*, was designed based on formative and summative evaluations to improve the knowledge, attitudes, and skills of interdisciplinary staff working with chronically mentally ill patients. The course featured active-directive training methods to convey the content areas of the curriculum identified above. Workshops were delivered in 15 states to over 1500 trainees. The following data illustrate the impact that the curriculum has had on students. Table 2 shows evaluative data obtained on participants' knowledge gained and attitudinal change in the workshop provided to over 100 psychiatry, psychology, social work, and nursing trainees from mental health facilities in the Los Angeles area who attended the 2-day workshop. Participants in this training experience also rated their satisfaction with the eight content

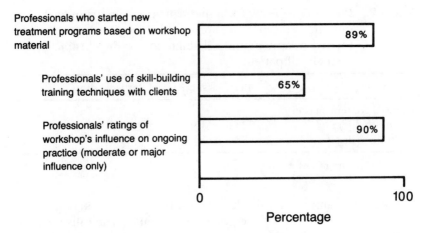

Figure 2. Six-month implementation of psychiatric rehabilitation methods by service providers.

areas covered. Ratings averaged 5 or above, on a 1–7 scale of satisfaction, for all content areas in terms of relevance of the material, informational value of the material, and interest level generated by the material. Follow-up utilization data from a similar presentation to interdisciplinary staff of state hospitals and community support programs from the states of Nebraska and Kansas are presented in Figure 2.

The true "test" of a training curriculum in psychiatric rehabilitation is not just trainee or student satisfaction, attitude change, or knowledge gain, but rather the actual utilization of the curriculum content with the chronically mentally ill. As indicated in Figure 2, the trainees did use the materials. The Community Support Program director for Nebraska reflected that the trainees viewed the workshop syllabus as their "bible" for "how to do" psychiatric rehabilitation. The Director of Mental Health for Kansas requested statewide treatment programming changes based on this curriculum. Although we cannot be sure of the fidelity of implementation of the treatment and rehabilitation methods reported by trainees attending this course, phone calls asking for specific technical assistance and follow-up communications from state mental health officials have increased our confidence in the actual utilization of these materials.

SUMMARY

Educational obstacles that must be overcome to provide education and training on the chronically mentally ill patient to all groups of professionals include the paucity of relevant curricula, the lack of interested, knowledgeable instructors, and the lag between research and practice, which is further amplified in the psychiatric rehabilitation area due to the comprehensive and complex nature of the intervention methods. A curriculum, *Psychiatric Rehabilitation of Chronic Mental Patients*, has been designed to overcome these obstacles. The curriculum features the stress-diathesis-coping-competence model of mental illness and principles of psychiatric rehabilitation in seven areas: 1) diagnostic and symptom-based assessment, 2) functional assessment and goal planning, 3) practical psychopharmacology, 4) social skills training techniques, 5) family education and communication skills training, 6) prevocational and vocational rehabilitation, and 7) comprehensive community support programs. The educational objectives of the curriculum are achieved through the use of active-directive training methods. It is not enough for trainees to acquire knowledge, experience, and positive attitudes toward the chronically mentally ill; behavioral skills are also required. Outcomes obtained from trainees exposed to the UCLA course from *Psychiatric Rehabilitation of Chronic Mental Patients* indicated that trainees were satisfied with the content, developed more positive attitudes toward the chronically mentally ill, experienced significant knowledge gains, and implemented the course content. This course is now part of the core curriculum for psychiatry residents at UCLA and is available as a text, a teacher's syllabus, and a video to use in graduate or professional education programs, workshops, and continuing education offerings.

REFERENCES

Backer TE, Liberman RP, Kuehnel TG: Dissemination and adoption of innovative psychosocial interventions. J Consult Clin Psychol 54:111–118, 1986

Brophy J: Teacher influences on student achievement. Am Psychol 41:1069–1072, 1986

Glaser EM, Abelson HH, Garrison KN: Putting Knowledge to Use. San Francisco, CA, Jossey-Bass, 1983

Hierholzer R, Liberman RP: Successful living: a social skills and problem-solving group for the chronic mentally ill. Hosp Community Psychiatry 37:913–918, 1986

Kane JM: Compliance issues in outpatient treatment. J Clin Psychopharmacol 5:22S–27S, 1985

Kuehnel TG, Flanagan SG: Training professionals: guidelines for effective continuing education workshops. The Behavior Therapist 1:5–8, 1984

Kuehnel TG, May PRA, Liberman RP: The zeitgeist of innovation: the road ahead. Knowledge: Creation, Diffusion, Utilization 8:270–273, 1986

Lefley HP, Cutler D: Training professionals to work with the chronically mentally ill. Community Ment Health J 24:253–257, 1988

Liberman RP (ed): Psychiatric Rehabilitation of Chronic Mental Patients. Washington, DC, American Psychiatric Press, 1987

Liberman RP, Phipps CC: Innovative techniques for the chronic mentally ill, in The Chronic Mental Patient/II. Edited by Menninger WW, Hannah G. Washington, DC, American Psychiatric Press, 1987

Liberman RP, Glynn S, Phipps CC: Rehabilitation of schizophrenic disorders, in Treatment of Psychiatric Disorders: A Task Force Report of the American Psychiatric Association, Vol 2. Washington, DC, American Psychiatric Press, 1989, pp 1567–1606

Matarazzo RG: Research on the teaching and learning of psychotherapeutic skills, in Handbook of Psychotherapy and Behavior Change: An Empirical Analysis, 2nd Edition. Edited by Garfield SL, Bergin AE. New York, John Wiley, 1978, pp 941–966

Meyerson AT: What are the barriers or obstacles to treatment and care of the chronically disabled mentally ill? in The Chronic Mental Patient: Problems, Solutions, and Recommendations for Public Policy. Edited by Talbott JA. Washington, DC, American Psychiatric Press, 1978

Mirabi M, Weinman ML, Magnetti SM, et al: Professional attitudes toward the chronic mentally ill. Hosp Community Psychiatry 36:404–405, 1985

Moore JD, David M: Staff Recruitment and Retention in Community Support Programs: A Ten State Study. Boulder, CO, Western Interstate Commission for Higher Education, 1984

Paul GL, Lentz RJ: Psychosocial Treatment of Chronic Mental Patients: Milieu Versus Social-Learning Programs. Cambridge, MA, Harvard University Press, 1977

Pepper B: The young adult chronic patient. J Clin Psychopharmacol 5:3S–7S, 1985

Search Institute: Principles for effecting needed change. Unpublished manuscript, Search Institute, 122 West Franklin, Suite 525, Minneapolis, MN 55404, 1984

Tupin JP: Focal neuroleptization: an approach for optimal dosing for initial and continuing therapy. J Clin Psychopharmacol 5:15S–21S, 1985

White HS, Bennett MB: Training psychiatric residents in chronic care. Hosp Community Psychiatry 32:339–343, 1981

Chapter 9

Functioning of Relatives and Patients Facing Severe Mental Illness

Shirley Glynn, Ph.D.
Robert Paul Liberman, M.D.

A conceptual framework for organizing the major points made in the chapters of this volume may be helpful in fostering a constructive dialogue and collaboration between mental health professionals and relatives of the mentally ill. The authors of the chapters in this book, most of them both professional persons and relatives of a mentally ill person, have cogently stated that

1. Having a mentally ill relative places an extraordinary, unremitting stress on all other family members.
2. Mental health professionals have failed, until recently, to offer beneficial services to families that are based on mutual respect and an absence of "blaming."
3. A comprehensive range of community-based mental health and rehabilitation services can support and reinforce the considerable coping efforts of relatives of the mentally ill.
4. Relatives and professionals can ally themselves in training other relatives and professionals to grasp the importance of a nonpejorative and sympathetic view of the noxious impact of mental illness on the family unit.

We are ready to develop a conceptual framework that integrates what is known about the determinants and process of functioning of both patients and relatives. The success of family organizations, spear-headed by the National Alliance for the Mentally Ill (NAMI), in shar-ing information, providing mutual support, and advocating for improved treatment and research in mental illness has magnified the coping resources of individual family members. Innovations in family-based interventions have equipped relatives and patients alike with the knowledge and skills necessary to deal with the stress of major mental illness in order to avoid relapse and to improve quality of life (Falloon et al. 1984, 1985; Anderson et al. 1986; Strachan 1986). A conceptual framework can provide clinicians and relatives with a means to address the multitude of issues that families must face and to gen-erate and test new hypotheses and treatments for family functioning.

The conceptual framework we will sketch views the experience of a severe and chronic mental disorder as an unfolding, reverberating process that extends over long periods of time. The process inter-twines patient and relatives in an embrace of stressful and protective factors that, combined with more enduring vulnerability factors, de-termines course and outcome for patient and relatives alike. The framework is depicted in Figure 1, with vulnerability, stress, and pro-tective factors diagramed separately for patients and relatives. The intermediate states that result when stressors, superimposed on vul-nerability, exceed the coping and protective resources available com-prise similar overarousal and stress experiences for patients and relatives. In contrast, variations in psychobiological vulnerability result in thresholds for experiencing stress that may be vastly different for patients and relatives. In addition, the outcomes—in emotional, phys-ical, vocational, and social domains—will usually be very different for patient as compared with relatives.

The stress-vulnerability-protective framework has been described in terms of the course and outcome of major mental disorders ex-perienced by patients (Zubin and Spring 1977; Liberman et al. 1980; Nuechterlein and Dawson 1984a; Anthony and Liberman 1986). Vul-nerability factors in patients are thought to be genetically mediated processes—such as central nervous system neurotransmitter abnor-malities and cognitive impairments—that are enduring over time with little amenability to change. Vulnerabilities are present before the first episode of illness and during periods of remission as well as relapse. Stressors that impinge on vulnerable individuals and precipitate or exacerbate psychopathology can include major life events, such as termination with a therapist, discharge from a hospital, or loss of a job.

The course and outcome of mental disorders depends also on the availability of protective factors that can buffer, neutralize, or compensate for stress and vulnerability. For example, a person with

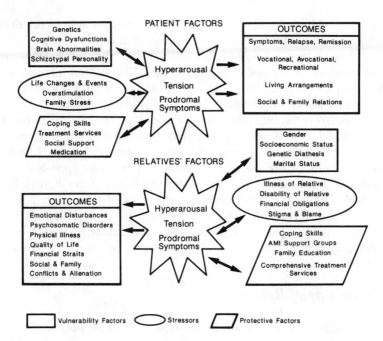

Figure 1. Conceptual framework for understanding factors involved in determining outcomes accruing to patients and relatives dealing with severe and chronic mental disorders.

schizophrenia who has good social skills and who can sustain a supportive set of relationships with relatives, friends, and treatment agencies will have a better outcome than a person lacking such skills (Liberman 1982). Antipsychotic medications, e.g., neuroleptics for schizophrenia and lithium for bipolar disorder, can serve as powerful protective bulwarks against stressors that inevitably arise in community life. In designing treatments for patients with major mental disorders, a focus on the protective factors can yield useful new interventions.

STRESS-VULNERABILITY-PROTECTIVE FACTORS IN RELATIVES

The stress-vulnerability-protective framework can be expanded and revised to include many critical issues for relatives of the mentally ill. This extension highlights the needs of all family members for constructive and supportive interventions from mental health professionals. Vulnerability for relatives resides in their sociodemographic status and in their own psychobiological diathesis. Stressors for relatives include the relapse of their sick family member, loss of financial resources, and blaming attitudes of mental health professionals. Protection from stress and vulnerability can derive from mutual support groups within the Alliance for the Mentally Ill (AMI), improved services from a local community mental health center, and respite housing in cases where the mentally ill person is living at home.

When stressors and vulnerability outweigh protective factors, family members will enter into a state of hyperarousal and stress. If unremitting, this high level of stress can have a deleterious impact on the family's quality of life, social adaptation, mental state, physical condition, and financial status, as described by Johnson in Chapter 2 of this book. Thus, the functioning of every family member, patient included, is determined by various biological, behavioral, and environmental forces that are constantly in flux; adaptive family functioning is associated with a surplus of protective factors over and above stress and vulnerability factors.

Vulnerability of Relatives

Investigations on the determinants of psychological well-being indicate that gender, marital status, and socioeconomic status all have a significant impact on quality of life. Unmarried women of low income or education are especially vulnerable to dysphoria and distress (Kessler 1979). Moreover, having previous history of psychiatric illness predisposes one to greater levels of psychological distress (Kessler et al. 1985). Studies have consistently found that women in the childbearing stage of their lives are particularly susceptible to depression, especially if they lack the protection that comes from having a close confidant in a relative or friend (Brown and Harris 1978).

In addition to the above-mentioned personal variables, vulnerability in a small percentage of relatives can come from a coinherited biological diathesis. Although less than 1% of the general population is at risk for schizophrenia, the risk based on genetic relationship is about 4–6% for parents, 8–10% for siblings, and 12–14% for offspring (Gottesman 1978). A small number of first-degree relatives of persons with schizophrenia have exhibited deficits in cognitive tasks requiring the processing of large amounts of information (e.g., vigilance, serial recall, span of apprehension) (Neuchterlein and Dawson 1984b). Hyperresponsivity and/or slow habituation to mildly aversive stimuli have also been noted in the psychophysiology of some offspring of schizophrenic patients (Dawson and Neuchterlein 1984). In interpreting these findings, however, it is important to note that most relatives performed no differently than control subjects, and there is no indication of a relationship to higher-order cognitive functioning.

However, the wide array of subtle deficits in some relatives may pre-dispose them to cognitive overload, hyperarousal, and stress-induced emotional or physical disorders.

Stressors Affecting Relatives

One of the most important sources of stress for relatives comes from the ups and downs of the illness in the sick family member— episodes of hospitalization, homelessness, vagrancy, psychotic symp-toms, and associated social and vocational disabilities. These stressors have been graphically and poignantly described in other chapters of this book as well as in books written by relatives (Walsh 1985; Hinckley et al. 1985) and professionals (Bernheim and Lehman 1985; Torrey 1988). Schizophrenia in a family member presents relatives with enor-mous challenges to understand, react, contain, and cope. Both positive and negative symptoms of the disorder—inappropriate or bizarre behavior, tenaciously held false beliefs, suspiciousness and unfounded fears, extreme social withdrawal and loss of initiative, unpredictable irritability, and even aggression—combine to pose a continuing bur-den of stress on the family unit.

With the scarce resources available for care of the chronically and severely mentally ill, families assume a disproportionate share of re-sponsibility for monitoring and supervision of their sick relatives. Vacations go by the board and interruptions in nighttime sleep be-come commonplace. One family, for example, experienced the great-est stressor from their schizophrenic son's coming into their bedroom and waking them to discuss his delusional fears and hallucinations.

Another source of stress comes from the heightened economic responsibility that having a nonworking young adult in the household produces. Social security benefits are unequal to the costs of main-taining a person in the community when that person incurs costs of medication, physician visits, and recurrent hospitalizations. Families low on the socioeconomic scale are especially vulnerable to this sort of stressor, as research has shown that poorer families actually ex-perience more aversive events and have fewer resources to cope with financial pressures (Kessler 1979). Even affluent families encounter difficulties in meeting the financial burden of a severely and chron-ically mentally ill relative (Johnson, Chapter 2, this book).

The community in which the patient and family live can also contribute to stress. For example, cutbacks in mental health services generally result in the family having more of the care-giving burden thrust on them. In one California county, agency staff reductions forced the closing of the mobile emergency team, which resulted in families having no responsive professionals, except the police, to call on for crisis services. Judgmental and stigmatizing cultural norms can also be stressful for families of the mentally ill. When the mentally ill are rejected by a community (e.g., by neighbors complaining about the opening of a residential care facility for the mentally ill), the family of the patient also experiences rejection. A society that, in effect, blames patients and their relatives for having a mental disorder is clearly exerting stress on the caring family (Hatfield 1978; Lefley 1989).

Protective Factors for Relatives

Being able to cope with the stressors impinging on a family harboring a mentally ill person is a major source of protection for relatives at risk for emotional, physical, social, and financial adversities. What, then, are the contributors to a family's coping ability? Having information about the nature of the illness and its treatment, developing realistic expectations for the functional capacities of the patient, using effective communication and problem-solving skills in everyday interactions, and obtaining and sustaining a collaborative relationship with professional care givers are all tributaries of successful coping (Hatfield 1978; Spiegel and Wissler 1986; Imber-Mintz et al. 1987).

Although it is not a simple task to recover from dashed hopes and unfulfilled dreams which relatives face as they grasp the serious, long-term illness of a family member (Kanter 1985), surviving schizophrenia or other chronic, recurring mental illnesses can be facilitated by practical and accessible forms of education provided by professionals (Anderson et al. 1986; Bernheim and Lewine 1979; Torrey 1988). The importance of effective problem solving in enhancing the lives of family members cannot be overemphasized. Effective resolution of life problems—stemming from the mentally ill relative or from stressors extrinsic to the family—can protect quality of life for all family members, just as poor problem solving by relatives can lead to increased stress and depression (Nezu and Ronan 1985). At the Clinical Research Center for Schizophrenia and Psychiatric Rehabilitation, Liberman and Falloon designed, implemented, and evaluated a structured and systematic program for teaching patients and relatives how to solve problems in living (Falloon and Liberman 1983; Falloon et al. 1984). This program was found, in carefully controlled research, to produce significant improvements in family functioning, relatives' psychological distress, and perceived burden in dealing with the sick family member.

Another important protective factor comes from the availability of comprehensive, long-term, and affordable treatment and rehabilitation programs for the mentally ill. Relatives are dependent on the care-giving system to provide housing, vocational rehabilitation, crisis intervention, case management, social skills training, medication services, and medical care for their sick family member. When these services are provided in a community, relatives are spared the inexorable stress associated with having primary care-giving responsibilities "dumped" into their laps.

Two other sources of coping are the social support networks established in many communities through AMI and the availability of social roles for the sick family member to fill within the family and the community. Whereas community attitudes of neglect and stigma toward the mentally ill can create stress for relatives, advocacy and mutual help through AMI groups can "buffer" the family from stress and improve overall functioning. The more favorable long-term prognosis for schizophrenia in underdeveloped and rural societies (Liberman 1982) may derive from extended, supportive kin networks and matter-of-fact attitudes toward mental illness, which foster functional reintegration into the community by the mentally ill, thereby adding hope and reducing burden on the immediate family (Lefley 1985; Leff 1981; Leff and Vaughn 1985).

PRODROMES OF DYSFUNCTIONAL OUTCOMES IN RELATIVES

The confluence of vulnerability, stress, and protective factors, shown in Figure 1 in the form of an interaction, can yield either good or poor outcomes for relatives and patients. When vulnerability and stress factors outweigh protective factors, hyperarousal and overload will be experienced and, unless reversed through intervention, may eventuate in psychological, social, and physical distress and symptoms. The relapse of a sick relative, the closing of a residential care facility, the unemployment of the family breadwinner, or a cut in social security benefits can all tip the balance toward a prodromal arousal state and subsequent dysfunction.

Some unfortunate families, bereft of coping and financial resources, may find themselves in an almost constant state of overarousal and tension; families with more protective resources would experience these prodromal periods briefly, albeit recurrently, and would be able to rapidly reestablish emotional equilibrium. However, even the most protected families would occasionally be exposed to prodromal periods of heightened tension. Recent surveys indicated that most relatives of the mentally ill experience reduced levels of life satisfaction at least part of the time (Johnson, Chapter 2, this book; Lefley 1987a).

EMOTIONAL, PHYSICAL, AND SOCIAL OUTCOMES
ACCRUING TO RELATIVES

Whether the overarousal and tension, depicted as intermediate states, lead to favorable or unfavorable outcomes depends on the balance of vulnerability, stress, and protective factors among the family members. Although outcomes are changing and dynamic, rather than static, they can be conveniently distributed into emotional, physical, and social domains. Living with a mentally ill person is an inherently painful, frustrating experience. First-person accounts are particularly poignant (Hinckley et al. 1985; Wechsler et al. 1988). Relatives of the mentally ill report higher levels of anxiety, depression, fear, anger, and psychosomatic ills than do nonrelatives (Arey and Warheit 1980). They also experience a wide variety of somatic complaints—headaches, gastrointestinal ailments, and worsening of medical disorders (Grad and Sainsbury 1968).

Siblings of the mentally ill, aware of the genetic transmission of disorders, worry about the possibility that they themselves or their children might develop mental illness. Because schizophrenia typically develops in late adolescence or early adulthood, parents find their plans for retirement or career change imperiled. Just as parents may be happily anticipating spending more time together, their child becomes a dependent adult with no prospect of early relief from the newly added burdens of close supervision. Marital relationships, sibling ties, and the quality of family life can be strained to the limit (Lefley 1987a).

Because of the stigma of mental illness, some families retreat from their previous social contacts and organizational involvements. Financial strain is almost inevitable; for example, an average of $44,000 spent on hospitalizations and treatment over a period of years is not atypical (Lefley 1987b). The symptoms and strains experienced by families, unless balanced by successful family coping and accessible community-based treatment and rehabilitation, can readily lead to disabilities in the relatives as well as in the patient.

The conceptual model also highlights the reciprocity between the major domains of influence. Having an enduring, affluent, and secure financial income may insulate and protect a family from problems; however, a sudden loss of income could immediately be a source of stress. A family that actively participates in the supportive program of an AMI chapter and then moves to another area where no such organizations exist can rapidly exchange a protective for a stress factor. Coping skills protect, but lifelong deficiencies in coping can create a kind of enduring, psychosocial vulnerability.

Partnership Between Relatives and Professionals

What, then, are the implications of the conceptual framework described above? One clear caveat is that treatment and rehabilitation for the patient can also be viewed as primary prevention of disorders in the relatives. To the extent that a comprehensive array of services is available to the patient, relatives are less likely to suffer adverse emotional and medical costs. A second implication lies in the interactions between the clinical status of the patient and the stress or protective factors affecting the relatives. The exacerbations of symptoms in a patient can lead directly to an increased stress load on the relatives, as can be seen in Figure 1. If the family has not been adequately educated by professionals regarding the nature and treatment of the disorder, unrealistic expectations, doubts about the legitimacy of the illness, and high levels of tension evoked by strange behavior could readily lead to the stress syndrome labeled "high expressed emotion." Unless supportive and other educational interventions are offered to the family, this high expressed emotion can provoke relapses in the patient (Vaughn et al. 1984). Similarly, treatment options should be made available to the relatives; for instance, catharsis, information giving, advice on "survival skills," and training in communication and problem solving can all be helpful in meeting the needs of relatives.

Summary

The conceptual framework for understanding both relatives' and patients' efforts to cope with major mental disorder can be useful for clinicians, researchers, and families. It offers an orientation for supportive and educational family interventions that acknowledges the needs of relatives for symptom relief and stress management. Possibilities for primary prevention of emotional disorders in relatives are viewed as interconnected with the availability of treatment and rehabilitation services for the patient. Research needs to be conducted on the variables—and their interaction—in the framework. For example, if some relatives have subtle cognitive dysfunctions because of genetic diatheses to a major mental disorder, how might interventions be designed to assist the relatives to overcome this liability? Similarly, if low socioeconomic status predisposes families to greater dysfunction, but coping can be enhanced through participation in support groups such as NAMI, how can support groups be made more accessible to poorer, less educated families? We hope that this model will generate research and intensive collaborative work among mental health professionals and the families of the mentally ill with the goal of improving the quality of life for all persons—family members and patients—affected by mental illness.

REFERENCES

Anderson CM, Reiss DJ, Hogarty GE: Schizophrenia in the Family: A Practitioner's Guide to Psychoeducation and Management. New York, Guilford, 1986

Anthony WA, Liberman RP: The practice of psychiatric rehabilitation. Schizophr Bull 12:542–559, 1986

Arey S, Warheit GJ: Psychosocial costs of living with psychologically disturbed family members, in The Social Consequences of Psychiatric Illness. Edited by Robins L, Wing JK. New York, Brunner/Mazel, 1980, pp 158–175

Bernheim KF, Lehman AF: Working With Families of the Mentally Ill. New York, WW Norton, 1985

Bernheim K, Lewine RRJ: Schizophrenia: Symptoms, Causes, Treatments. New York, WW Norton, 1979

Brown GW, Harris TO: Social Origins of Depression: A Study of Psychiatric Disorder in Women. London, Tavistock, 1978

Dawson ME, Neuchterlein KH: Psychophysiological dysfunctions in the developmental course of schizophrenic disorders. Schizophr Bull 10:204–232, 1984

Falloon IRH, Liberman RP: Behavioral family interventions in the management of chronic schizophrenia, in Family Therapy of Schizophrenia. Edited by McFarlane W. New York, Guilford, 1983, pp 117–137

Falloon IRH, Boyd JL, McGill CW: Family Care of Schizophrenia. New York, Guilford, 1984

Falloon IRH, Boyd JL, McGill CW, et al: Family management in the prevention of morbidity of schizophrenia. Arch Gen Psychiatry 42:887–896, 1985

Goldman HH, Gatozzi AA: Defining and counting the chronically mentally ill. Hosp Community Psychiatry 32:21–27, 1981

Gottesman II: Schizophrenia and genetics: Where are we? Are you sure? in The Nature of Schizophrenia: New Approaches to Research and Treatment. Edited by Wynne LC, Cromwell RL, Matthysse S. New York, John Wiley, 1978, pp 59–69

Grad J, Sainsbury P: The effects that patients have on their families in a community care and a control psychiatric service: a two year follow-up. Br J Psychiatry 114:265–278, 1968

Hatfield AB: Psychological costs of schizophrenia to the family. Social Work 23:355–359, 1978

Hinckley J, Hinckley J, Sherrill E: Breaking Points. Grand Rapids, MI, Chosen Books, 1985

Imber-Mintz L, Liberman RP, Miklowitz D, et al: Expressed emotion: a clarion call for a partnership between relatives and professionals. Schizophr Bull 13:227–235, 1987

Kanter JS: Talking with families about coping strategies, in Clinical Issues in Treating the Chronic Mentally Ill (New Directions for Mental Health Services No 27). Edited by Kanter JS. San Francisco, CA, Jossey-Bass, 1985, pp 7–19

Kessler RC: Stress, social status, and psychological distress. J Health Soc Behav 20:259–272, 1979

Kessler RC, Price RH, Wortman CB: Social factors in psychopathology: stress, social support, and coping processes. Ann Rev Psychol 36:531–572, 1985

Leff J: Psychiatry Around the Globe: A Transcultural View. New York, Marcel Dekker, 1981

Leff J, Vaughn C: Expressed Emotion in Families: Its Significance for Mental Illness. New York, Guilford, 1985

Lefley HP: Families of the mentally ill in cross cultural perspective. Psychosocial Rehabilitation Journal 8:57–75, 1985

Lefley HP: Aging parents as caregivers of mentally ill adult children: an emerging social problem. Hosp Community Psychiatry 38:1063–1070, 1987a

Lefley HP: Impact of mental illness in families of mental health professionals. J Nerv Ment Dis 175:613–619, 1987b

Lefley HP: Family burden and family stigma in major mental illness. Am Psychol 44:556–560, 1989

Liberman RP: Social factors in the etiology of the schizophrenic disorders, in Psychiatry 1982: The American Psychiatric Association Annual Review, Vol 1. Edited by Grinspoon L. Washington, DC, American Psychiatric Press, 1982, pp 97–112

Liberman RP, Wallace CJ, Vaughn CE, et al: Social and family factors in the course of schizophrenia: toward an interpersonal problem solving therapy for schizophrenics and their relatives, in Psychotherapy of Schizophrenia: Current Status and New Directions. Edited by Strauss J, Fleck S, Bowers M, et al. New York, Plenum, 1980

Neuchterlein KH, Dawson ME: A hueristic vulnerability/stress model of schizophrenic episodes. Schizophr Bull 10:300–312, 1984a

Neuchterlein KH, Dawson ME: Information processing and attentional functioning in the developmental course of schizophrenic disorders. Schizophr Bull 10:160–203, 1984b

Nezu AM, Ronan GF: Life stress, current problems, problem solving, and depressive symptoms: an integrative model. J Consult Clin Psychol 53:693–697, 1985

Spiegel D, Wissler T: Family environment as a predictor of psychiatric hospitalization. Am J Psychiatry 143:56–60, 1986

Strachan AM: Family intervention for the rehabilitation of schizophrenia: toward protection and coping. Schizophr Bull 12:678–698, 1986

Torrey EF: Surviving Schizophrenia: A Family Manual, Revised Edition. New York, Harper & Row, 1988

Vaughn CE, Snyder KS, Jones S, et al: Family factors in schizophrenic relapse. Arch Gen Psychiatry 41:1169–1177, 1984

Walsh M: Schizophrenia: Straight Talk for Families and Friends. New York, Morrow, 1985

Wechsler JA, Schwartztol HW, Wechsler NF: In a Darkness: A Story of Young Suicide, 2nd Edition. Miami, FL, Pickering Press, 1988

Zubin J, Spring B: Vulnerability—a new view of schizophrenia. J Abnorm Psychol 86:103–126, 1977

Guidelines for Working With Families of the Chronically Mentally Ill

Christine McGill, Ph.D.

Two themes that have emerged from the family consumer movement are the recognition of the salutary effects of family empowerment (Battaglino 1987) through advocacy efforts of the National Alliance for the Mentally Ill (NAMI) and the need to rectify the sins of the past in order to establish collaborative partnerships between families and mental health professionals (Johnson 1987). Historically, mental health professionals have been wary of involvement with consumer groups and have easily become defensive in response to criticisms leveled at prevailing mental health treatment resources.

More recently, mental health professionals have begun to acknowledge the positive impact of consumer activity in advocating for more resources. Innovative treatment models such as the coping-competence paradigm described in the preceding chapter have given rise to new optimism about future collaborative relationships between families and mental health professionals. However, this must be tempered by the recognition of certain grim realities; namely, that available mental health services for the chronically disabled remain woefully inadequate and unavailable to families, thus constituting a major family stressor. Families continue to come up against negative attitudes from mental health professionals in many settings (McElroy 1987). The burden placed on families to provide care for their mentally ill relative remains enormous. An explicit goal of any intervention involving families must be the amelioration of the manifest burden. Few guidelines or instruments are available to clinicians to assess the level of family burden. In applying a stress-diathesis coping-competence model to the functioning of relatives, we need to focus on identification of stressors that are remediable and target psychosocial strategies to reduce the stress associated with them. What I am struck by in the conceptual framework so elegantly presented by Glynn and Liberman is that all of the relatives' stressors relate to the broader construct of family burden and attitudes toward illness, and that no factors extrinsic to the family are identified except for societal stigma, which is patient related and affects all members of the family. Another puzzling aspect of this schema is that life events and family stress are viewed as patient stressors when in fact their effects can be deleterious to family members as well. A more meaningful distinction in assessing family stressors may be the degree of patient relatedness.

The burden of living with a person with a chronic illness has been well described in these pages. For many families, there is the fond recollection of the way things were before the person became ill, and how things were supposed to be, versus the painful reality of the current level of disability. This discrepancy in functioning is heightened by the accomplishments of siblings and friends. The patient's pain about the illness and the limitations that it places on him or her are crosses that the entire family must bear. Furthermore, many patients distort or deny their illness and project their problems onto family members. Absolution from guilt is a long-term process for many families even when they have accepted the fact that etiologically they are not to blame. Having a child with a defect, albeit biological, is difficult to accept without remorse.

Several additional factors have been implicated as contributing to severe burden of family care givers. Elderly parents are often unable to handle the demands for care placed on them by their chronically ill and dependent sons or daughters (Lefley 1987a). Single parents without family support are similarly at risk to be the patient's total support system. Thurer (1983) and Lefley (1987b) have suggested that community care of the chronically disabled is a women's issue because of the traditional female care-giving role taking precedence over career aspiration. Poverty and overcrowding frequently are ongoing stressors or enduring characteristics that raise family burden beyond tolerable limits.

Thus, it may be concluded that families caring for a mentally ill relative suffer considerable hardship in the majority of cases. The range of burden may vary from mild to severe, with many families struggling valiantly to cope with a severely impaired family member in the absence of professional support. One has to question the wisdom of using the family as a resource for provision of round-the-clock skilled nursing care.

Understandably, many families suffer from burnout much the same as that reported by mental health workers in acute settings. Despite the recognition of this phenomenon, the concept of respite care remains elusive as a resource to families providing chronic care in the community.

ASSESSMENT OF STRESSORS

Because we are focusing on educating mental health professionals to work with the families of the chronically mentally ill, I would like to suggest some guidelines for the assessment of family stressors and burden, which can be ameliorated by supportive empathic intervention on the part of clinicians. First and foremost, we must listen to families and acknowledge our respect for their care-giving efforts. We must learn to accept that their pain and burden are normal coping responses to dealing with their psychiatrically impaired family member and that they do not harbor an investment in the patient's dysfunction. Their distress should not be construed as evidence of family disturbance, which then becomes labeled as individual psychopathology. The delineation of the diathesis-stress-coping factors in relatives as distinct from those of patients is important and may present a treatment dilemma to the clinician. Hatfield indicated in Chapter 3 of this book that patient needs and family needs are not necessarily congruent, and that working with relatives and patients requires acknowledgment of these differences in terms of conflict resolution through compromise.

Although it is important for the clinician to be aware of vulnerability factors in family members, the focus of treatment lies in stress reduction. Thus, identification of family stressors as well as family strengths is of paramount importance. Clinicians need to acknowledge positive family coping and start with the assumption that families are doing the best they can to cope with a difficult situation. In examining stressors in relation to depression, a distinction has been made between life events and major difficulties (Brown and Harris 1978). Major difficulties were defined as enduring characteristics that persisted over time and were of an unpleasant nature. Caring for a schizophrenic or chronically mentally ill relative was one such major difficulty. Others included problems in the areas of employment, housing, health, childrearing, marriage, social obligations, friends, leisure, money, neighborhood, and general disappointment. Major difficulties and life events such as loss or separation could bring about depression either independently or in combination. Thus, stressors or problems in living that are unrelated to the patient with schizophrenia need to be taken into account. They may be external to the family, such as school problems and job dissatisfaction, or they may have to do with relationships within the family.

In multiproblem families, the patient's illness may be just one of many stressors, including poverty, substance abuse, and involvement with the criminal justice system. In any event, the degree of perceived patient relatedness of problems is of major importance in family assessment. Where there is much distress around the ill family member's role performance and/or social functioning, families will report considerable burden associated with care-giving activity. The stressors on families outlined in the conceptual model described in Figure 1 of the preceding chapter—the illness and disability of the relative, financial obligations, stigma and blame—are all aspects of the broader concept of family burden.

The assumption of family burden can be made a priori in most cases where the impairment from functional psychiatric illness is substantial. The concept of family burden originates from the breakdown of reciprocity in family relationships, so that parents, spouses, or siblings of mentally ill family members are saddled with disproportionate responsibility for their care. This arrangement may place restrictions on the activities or life-style of all family members. Social expectations are highly variable and difficult to measure, making individual family assessment important in shaping subsequent intervention. Many families have difficulty with adjustment of patient expectations, especially where premorbid functioning was high. Even when expectations are realistically set, frustration with low social functioning may ensue. Few instruments have been developed to assess family burden, although one such measure, the Social Behavior Assessment Schedule, was developed in England for this purpose. It is a semistructured interview conducted with a relative, which attempts to quantify both objective and subjective burden over a 3-month period. The interview has utility as a research tool in that the amount of burden can be assessed repeatedly to measure how families are coping over time (Platt et al. 1980). Standard areas of inquiry that are clinically relevant in evaluating family burden include amount of objective and subjective distress experienced by the family. Although much of this burden is usually related to the patient's illness, some aspects may be unrelated, or the degree of relatedness may be unclear. For example, an elderly parent's poor health may impose restrictions on socialization outside the home, independent of the patient's illness. However, the patient's illness may exacerbate the care giver's health status. The likelihood of objective burden increases the longer the patient remains ill (Hoenig and Hamilton 1966; Noh and Turner 1987).

The following are indices of objective burden commonly reported by relatives, which clinicians need to assess.

1. *Financial hardship*: loss of wages or time off from work of family members; foregone wages of the ill family member; loss of entitlements such as social security income, Veterans Administration benefits, and medical assistance, or failure to apply for such benefits; amount of financial support provided by the family for the ill member with no available resources.
2. *Health*: physical illness; anxiety, depression, worry.
3. *Restriction of social and leisure activity*: disruption of household routine; isolation from friends, neighbors, family; no vacations; discomfort in leaving the patient; amount of activity outside of the home.

Concomitant with the presence of objective family burden, there is often subjective distress or dissatisfaction that may reflect individual coping style. Subjective burden has been defined as the extent to which family members report feeling burdened by the illness. Both the amount of distress or dissatisfaction with the patient's behavior and whether the patient's role dysfunction is seen as illness related are important dimensions to assess. The construct of expressed emotion (EE), which measures criticality, hostility, and emotional involvement of relatives, is really tapping the family's perception of the patient's symptoms and illness behavior that are burdensome and distressing. The EE rating per se is a gross measure of the family's account of the current level of stress and tension around the patient's illness. If the level of family burden is high, then the affective climate or EE may be quite tense. The clinician must acknowledge both the presence of tension in sessions and the benefits of lowering this stress level in daily living. Family assessment of subjective burden can be measured by probing the following areas:

1. What are the family's knowledge and attitudes about the patient's illness?
2. What are the most bothersome behaviors and symptoms?
3. How do they cope with them?
4. How much tension does the patient's illness generate?
5. How do they see the future?
6. What helps?
7. What makes things worse?

8. What do they think would be helpful in terms of treatment now?
9. How much time do they spend in direct contact with the patient?
10. What are the individual goals unrelated to the patient of family members?

In a stress-diathesis-coping model, it is essential that the clinician acknowledge the objective family burden in a supportive, empathic way, be prepared to offer referrals for resources, and give direct advice. To assess the more subtle subjective burden, the clinician must elicit specific information from the family's perspective on the above-mentioned areas. This is best accomplished in brief individual interviews with each family member, as individual perceptions may vary widely. Based on the input from family members, the clinician can plan treatment strategies to meet the family's needs. The clinician may initiate the family sessions by summarizing the content provided in individual interviews and by formally identifying family coping strengths. These may include recognition of the patient's illness or symptoms, seeking treatment for the patient, recognition of the importance of medication, provision of resources, etc.

Because families may be wary of the clinician's agenda initially, it is imperative that the conceptual framework of stress, vulnerability, and coping be spelled out as part of the treatment contract. Many families will need continued reassurance that the goal in working with family members is in fact enhanced coping, and that there is no covert agenda to correct "pathological" relationships. Family members may have good reason to question the appropriateness of family intervention based on prior negative treatment experiences. Inquiry about past exposure to mental health professionals often yields information that will serve to further sensitize the clinician to the family's plight in dealing with the mental health system.

STRATEGIES TO HELP FAMILIES COPE WITH STRESSORS

Families who have had involvement with NAMI or a psycho-educational program are often quite knowledgeable about their family member's illness. However, they may still have difficulty coping with more subtle aspects of the disability, such as the negative symptoms. If family members do not understand their relative's schizophrenia or affective illness, this is a good place to start. Clinicians should endeavor to tailor their intervention to the family's need for information and level of comprehension. Educational material is best presented repeatedly over time. While an all-day workshop may be stimulating and beneficial in terms of engendering support among family members, it may amount to sensory overload if too much new information is presented. This has led some investigators to note that relatives remember only a small amount of what is reviewed in educational sessions (Berkowitz et al. 1984). Tarrier and Barrowclough (1986) hypothesize that relatives develop a lay model of schizophrenia over time, which they bring into educational sessions and which influences their acceptance or rejection of new information. The longer the patient has been ill, the less receptive family members are likely to be to changing their belief systems. Difficulties in changing family beliefs and attitudes may have been underestimated by previous investigators (Hogarty et al. 1986; McGill et al. 1983). The importance of family educational intervention early in the course of schizophrenic disorder should be underscored.

Core topics for discussion in most educational interventions have included diagnosis, symptoms, etiology, epidemiology, popular myths, medication, course and prognosis, and treatment and management issues. Preferably, symptoms and course can be described in terms of the patient's individual presentation. Identification of prodromal signs of relapse are likewise idiosyncratic to the patient and need to be elicited from the patient and the family. Whenever possible, the patient needs to be engaged as the expert on his or her illness. Debating etiology with family members is often counterproductive. I have known several parents, highly educated with advanced degrees in the behavioral sciences, who believe steadfastly that schizophrenia is caused by childhood developmental problems and aspects of their parenting. Both have sons in their forties who have been chronically institutionalized for severe "process" schizophrenia. Rather than trying to influence them with alternative explanations, I have conceded to our different perspectives on causation and stressed that agreement on aspects of diagnosis and treatment is more important. Similarly, it is not useful to challenge cultural beliefs about mental illness. Sometimes what is most effective is the simple acknowledgment that the causes of schizophrenia remain unknown.

Families have long identified their need for information and advice on symptom management. For many family members, identification of symptoms is perplexing, as is dealing with them consistently. For example, many well-intentioned relatives will cope with delusions by attempting to rationally dissuade the patient from believing in them. Others may laugh at the absurdity of such beliefs, ignore them, or openly challenge them. None of these coping strategies is particularly effective, and clinicians need to be prepared to give direct advice and model other strategies for dealing with symptoms. Family members should be encouraged to acknowledge empathically that the patient has particular false beliefs, at the same time pointing out that they do not share those beliefs themselves.

Family members can likewise learn to effectively set limits around difficult patient behaviors. Any efforts that are made to change noxious patterns need to be reviewed and supported by the clinician. For example, if the family is bothered by the patient's talking to himself or herself and this is an ongoing problem related to unremitting hallucinations, as it often is, the clinician has a number of important tasks: 1) to make sure the family understands the patient's behavior as a coping response to schizophrenic symptoms, 2) to request that the family tell the patient how the behavior is upsetting or embarrassing to them, 3) to encourage the family to come up with alternative coping strategies, and 4) to monitor their efforts over time.

Two potential strategies that are often useful for dealing with problem behaviors are time-outs and contracting. Families can ask that patients go to their rooms or stay away from family members while they respond to internal stimuli in order to reduce family stress. Rewards or reinforcement may be a successful means of decreasing bothersome behaviors, particularly negative symptoms like apathy and lack of activity. Family members are in the best position to identify reinforcers that the patient particularly likes, such as foods, personal items, or entertainment. If family members are reluctant to use such strategies or see it as "bribing" the patient, the clinician needs to be prepared to educate the family about the effectiveness of behavior techniques in the treatment of a wide range of problems including eating disorders, sexual dysfunction, phobias, etc. Often what families are really reacting to is the enormous dependency needs of their ill relative and the desire to encourage adult developmental norms such as independence, which are often not realistic given chronic psychotic illness.

Another strategy that can be quite effective in lowering family stress and tension is decreasing the amount of direct face-to-face contact that family members have with the ill relative. The British work on EE has suggested that lowering the amount of direct contact to under 35 hours a week may have advantages as a "protective" factor that lowers relapse rates (Leff et al. 1982). Patients and family members need support from the clinician to increase independent socialization. If family members are reticent about leaving the patient alone, use of problem solving to achieve this goal will be extremely useful. With many chronic problems, such as increasing social activity, the clinician must repeatedly deal with the same problem on a regular basis in a supportive manner. The clinician must resist the temptation to label the family as resistant merely because the same problems of daily living continue to emerge.

Most families of the chronically mentally ill will identify the burden associated with obtaining resources in a crisis and the lack of system responsiveness to families at times of hospitalization or emergency intervention. Families can often benefit from crisis telephone consultation on weekends and evenings. Programs that treat the severely mentally ill must be prepared to provide such backup services, which are sorely lacking at the community level. Clinicians also need to be prepared to establish liaison with psychiatric emergency facilities on behalf of families when that level of intervention is warranted.

Last, clinicians should routinely inform families of available self-help resources such as local Alliance for the Mentally Ill groups as part of sound clinical practice. Clinicians should subscribe to the monthly newsletter that most local groups mail to members and be aware of the time and location of share and care and support groups. It is important for clinicians to recognize the importance of peer support and empowerment in combating the effects of stigmatization, isolation, and loss of self-esteem which relatives suffer as a result of caring for their chronically ill family member.

SUMMARY

Clinicians working with the chronically mentally ill and their relatives have begun to embrace conceptual models that emphasize the combined efficacy of psychosocial and psychopharmacological interventions such as the stress-vulnerability-coping paradigm comprehensively outlined in the preceding chapter. They must be provided with the clinical tools to deliver such interventions. The clinician must first acknowledge that the needs of the patient and those of the family may be quite different. The clinician should be prepared to "treat" the patient for the mental disorder; however, the clinician should not assume that the family desires treatment, unless such a contract is explicit. The clinician needs to be available to collaborate with the family in a partnership that focuses on the management of the patient's illness with the assumption that stabilization of the illness will promote family well-being and vice versa. This calls for the clinician to be knowledgeable about the complexity of the mental disorder and its management in order to convey such expertise to relatives in a supportive context. In working with families, the framework needs to go beyond a "no fault" position to one that recognizes the enormous burden that families face in caring for a chronically ill member and how these many aspects of burden are manifested in families of varied socioeconomic and ethnic status. The clinician needs to be sensitive to the cumulative effects of patient burden, life events, and problems of daily living, both patient related and independent of the illness.

The goals in working with families should be directed at ameliorating both the objective and subjective burden experienced in most families, by enhancing coping through problem-solving efforts. Family strengths ought to be explicitly acknowledged in working with families, rather than focusing primarily on deficits. Clinicians must remember that all models have practical limitations, and when all else fails, the importance of maintaining a supportive respectful relationship with families, as well as with patients, cannot be emphasized strongly enough.

REFERENCES

Battaglino L: Family empowerment through self-help groups, in Families of the Mentally Ill: Meeting the Challenges, Vol 34. Edited by Hatfield AB. San Francisco, CA, Jossey-Bass, 1987, pp 43–52

Berkowitz R, Eberlein-Vries R, Kuipers L, et al: Educating relatives about schizophrenia. Schizophr Bull 7:418–429, 1984

Brown CW, Harris T: Social Origins of Depression. London, Tavistock, 1978

Hoenig J, Hamilton MW: The schizophrenic patient in the community and his effect on the household. Int J Soc Psychiatry 12:165–176, 1966

Hogarty GE, Anderson CM, Reiss DJ, et al: Family psychoeducation, social skills training, and maintenance chemotherapy in the aftercare treatment of schizophrenia. Arch Gen Psychiatry 43:633–642, 1986

Johnson DL: Professional-family collaboration, in Families of the Mentally Ill: Meeting the Challenges, Vol 34. Edited by Hatfield AB. San Francisco, CA, Jossey-Bass, 1987, pp 73–80

Leff J, Kuipers L, Berkowitz R, et al: A controlled trial of social intervention in the families of schizophrenic patients. Br J Psychiatry 141:121–134, 1982

Lefley HP: Aging parents as caregivers of mentally ill adult children: an emerging social problem. Hosp Community Psychiatry 38:1063–1070, 1987a

Lefley HP: The family's response to mental illness in a relative, in Families of the Mentally Ill: Meeting the Challenges, Vol 34. Edited by Hatfield AB. San Francisco, CA, Jossey-Bass, 1987b, pp 3–22

McElroy EM: Sources of distress among families of the hospitalized mentally ill, in Families of the Mentally Ill: Meeting the Challenges, Vol 34. Edited by Hatfield AB. San Francisco, CA, Jossey-Bass, 1987, pp 61–72

McGill CW, Falloon IRH, Boyd JL, et al: Family educational intervention in the treatment of schizophrenia. Hosp Community Psychiatry 34:934–938, 1983

Noh S, Turner RJ: Living with psychiatric patients: implications for the mental health of family members. Soc Sci Med 25:263–271, 1987

Platt S, Weyman A, Hirsch S, et al: The Social Behavior Assessment Schedule (SBAS): rationale, contents scoring and reliability of a new intervention schedule. Soc Psychiatry 15:43–55, 1980

Tarrier N, Barrowclough C: Providing information to relatives about schizophrenia: some comments. Br J Psychiatry 149:458–463, 1986

Thurer SL: Deinstitutionalization and women: where the buck stops. Hosp Community Psychiatry 34:1162–1163, 1983

Index

Advocacy. *See* Consumer advocacy
Alliance for the Mentally Ill (AMI) of
New York, 202–203, 205, 214
Alzheimer's disease, 128
American Psychiatric Association
(APA), response to
homosexuality, 82
Asylums
contemporary treatment
perspective, 13–14, 18–20, 26
family influence, 6–9, 10
historical perspective, 5–6, 11–12
provider-family relationships,
100–101
supportive aftercare, 14
Attribution theory, 137–138
Autism, 82–83

Beane v. McMullen, 177
Behavior management skills, 107
Biological roots of mental illness,
13, 102–103, 118
Board-and-care homes, 14, 26
Burden
Alzheimer's disease example, 128
assessing, 269–272
economic, 38–39, 259, 262
level of, 43–44, 268–269
minimizing, 55–57, 267
objective, 35–37, 271
subjective, 37–38, 271–272
See also Impact of mental illness
on family members
Burnout, 107–108, 269

Children of the mentally ill, 41–42
Chlorpromazine, 11

Chronicity
barrier to provider-family
relationship, 110–111
critical evaluation of data, 123
emphasizing professional reward
for treating, 122–123
exposure of professionals to
families, 120–121, 168
professionals, problems dealing
with, 116–117
support networks for
professionals, 121–122
training for, 117, 119, 168
understanding, 121, 167–168
Clinical Research Center for
Schizophrenia and Psychiatric
Rehabilitation, 250, 260
Collaborative discharge planning, 19
Columbia University School of
Social Work, 203–215
Communication
deviance, 140
importance in provider-family
relationship, 103–105
Community-based treatment
burden, 44–45
discharge from hospital, 17,
19–20
family responsibility, 12–13
historical perspective, 11–13
Confidentiality, 176–178, 195
See also Privacy
Consumer advocacy
approach to professional schools,
203–204
coping role, 152–153, 256, 261

development of NAMI, 84–86
disability-reduction role, 96–97
themes, 267
Contracting between provider and
    families, 197–198
Coping strategies
    burden minimizing role, 56–57
    consumer advocacy movement
        role, 152–153, 256, 261
    contributing factors, 260–261
    low EE in patient care, 151–152
    research on healthy family
        members, 150–151
    training, 106–107, 260
Corporate medicine, 87
Cost of services
    corporate medicine, 87
    estimate, 86
    medical insurance role, 86–87
Cross-cultural research issues
    Israeli High Risk Study, 143–144
    schizophrenia research, 142–143
    self-perception of families, 143
    value orientations impact, 143
    variables, 140, 142

Deinstitutionalization
    difficulties for patients, 19–20
    effects on families, 17, 44–45,
        125
    effects on mental health
        professionals, 242
    legal issues, 146–147
    social role issues, 145–146
Disability
    definition, 92
    family movement role in
        reducing, 96–97
    interaction of sources, 95–96
    primary, 92–93
    secondary, 93–94
    social pressure role, 94–95
    tertiary, 94
Dysfunctional families, 52–53, 261

Economic burden of mental illness,
    38–39, 259, 262
Education of mental health
    professionals
    curriculum orientations, 188
    impact of mental illness on
        family, 168, 198–200,
        201–215, 217–221

interviewing practices, 188–191
promoting new paradigms,
    201–215, 217–221
recommendations, 188–191,
    198–200
schizophrenia, 165–168
See also Fieldwork
EE. See Expressed emotion
Ethical issues
    confidentiality, 176–178
    family therapy research, 148–149
    interviewing practices, 180–181
    privacy of families, 177–178,
        179–181
    privacy of patients, 196
    professional organizations,
        187–188
    research issues, 147–149
Expressed emotion (EE)
    family reaction to patient
        behavior, 24, 271
    high- and low-EE families, 24–25
    research issues, 166–167
    and schizophrenia, 23–24,
        142–143, 274
    social implications of research,
        144–145

Family deviance
    "normal" deviance, 139–140
    research criteria, 138–139
    sources of stress model, 140
Family therapy
    historical perspective, 10–11
    iatrogenic effects, 134–135
    research ethics, 148–149
    UCLA Family Project, 15–16
Family training programs
    behavior management skills, 107
    burden minimizing role, 57
    problem-solving skills training,
        106–107, 260, 263
    stress management, 107
Fieldwork
    UCLA curriculum
        evaluation, 251–252
        goals, 244–247
        instruction methods,
            247–251
        obstacles, 242–244

University of Wisconsin
  curriculum
    agency benefits, 226–227
    attitudes of students,
      225–226
    competencies after one year,
      237–238
    goals, 227–228
    instruction methods,
      228–230
    obstacles, 224–226
    other assignments, 232–235
    placements, 230–231
    reading and writing
      assignments, 231–232
    student development,
      235–237

Gay Liberation Front, 81–82

Halfway houses, 14
Historical perspective
  asylums, 5–9
  community-based care, 11–13
  contemporary treatment, 13–20
  families of the mentally ill, 32–33
  psychoanalytic theories, 9–11
  reason for, 3
Hollander v. Lubow, 177
Homelessness among mentally ill,
  95–96
Homosexuals, negative response of
  mental health professionals,
  81–82
Hygosystogenic distress, 184–185

Iatrogenic distress
  conflicting messages, 133–135
  damage to family members, 132,
    164, 184
  damage to patients, 132–133
Impact of mental illness on family
  members
  assessing, 269–272
  attitudes toward families, 52–54,
    80–84, 100–101, 183–184,
    199–200, 267
  children, 41–42, 258
  conflict between professionals and
    family members, 52
  deinstitutionalization, 44–45, 125
  dysfunctional families, 52–53,
    261

economic burden, 38–39, 259, 262
  level of burden, 43–44
  mental health care providers,
    satisfaction with, 46–51,
    54–55
  minimizing, 55–57, 267
  objective burden, 35–37, 271
  outcomes, 261–262
  parents, 39–40, 262, 268
  relatives, 42–43, 258–260,
    261–262
  research issues, 164–165
  siblings, 40–41, 150, 262
  spouses, 40
  subjective burden, 37–38,
    271–272
  surveys, 34–35
  time consideration, 45
Informed consent
  components, 196
  contract model, 197–198
  defined, 176, 195
  education of mental health
    professionals, 188–191
  interviews, 176, 179–180, 196
  problems, 196–197
  recommendations, 190–191
Insurance, relation to cost of
  services, 86–87
Interviewing families
  case studies, 174–181
  coercive strategies, 182–185
  educating mental health
    professionals, 188–191
  family role in change, 185–188
  guidelines, 185
  hygosystogenic distress, 184–185
  retribution for noncompliance,
    181–182, 185
Israeli High Risk Study, 143–144

Joint Commission on Accreditation
  of Health Care Organizations
  (JCAHO), 17, 187

Least restrictive environment
  doctrine, 77–78
Legal issues
  barriers to provider-family
    relationship, 111
  invasion of privacy, 177–178

Level of burden
  assessing, 269–272
  deinstitutionalization, 44–45
  mental health professionals,
    46–51
  support networks, 45–46
  symptom level, 43–44
  time factor, 45
Life events research
  differential impact on family
    members, 130–131
  life events scales, 130
  normative life transitions and
    catastrophic life events, 130
  uneven course of psychotic illness
    role, 131
Lithium, 257

Manic-depression, biological roots,
    118
Medication
  informing families, 106
  monitoring by family, 109
  relevance of patient's response,
    118
Mental health professionals
  attitudes toward chronically ill,
    225–226, 242–243
  attitudes toward family members,
    52–54, 80–84, 100–101,
    183–184, 199–200, 267
  attitudinal changes,
    recommendations, 120–123,
    199–200
  burden minimizing role, 56–57,
    272–275
  chronicity, dealing with, 110–111,
    116–117
  conflict with family members, 52
  contradictions between
    professional ideas, 83
  family members, needs, 54–55,
    118
  iatrogenic effects of clinician's
    behavior, 131–138, 184
  negative response to
    homosexuals, 81–82
  negative response to women
    patients, 82
  nonmedical, 119
  surveys of families' reactions to,
    46–51
  See also Education of mental

health professionals;
  Provider-family relationship
Mental illness
  biological roots, 13
  impact on family members, 33–59
  major features, 33, 34
Mother-as-pathogen, 9–10

National Alliance for the Mentally
    Ill (NAMI)
  coping role, 152–153, 256, 258,
    261, 267
  deinstitutionalization position,
    145–146
  development, 33, 84–86
  family as caregivers position, 80
  self-help role, 107–108
National Society for Autistic
    Children, 82
Neuroleptics, 257

Objective burden of mental illness,
    35–37

Parents of the mentally ill, 39–40,
    262, 268
Primary disability, 92–93
Privacy
  education of mental health
    professionals, 188–191
  families' right to, 177–178,
    179–181
  patients' right to, 196
  recommendations, 190–191
Problem behavior strategies, 274
Protective factors for relatives,
    260–261, 274
  See also Coping strategies
Provider-family relationship
  asylum role, 100
  barriers, 110–111
  care-taking role of family,
    109–110
  chronicity barrier, 110–111,
    116–117, 119
  communication channels,
    103–105
  contracting, 197–198
  crisis consultation, 274–275
  decision-making role of family, 103
  education role of provider,
    105–106, 119–120, 263

families' observations and
    intuitions role, 108
family "burnout" recognition,
    107–108
family motivation, 101–103
family style, 103, 263
goals, 275–276
historical perspective, 3–20
ideal, 104–105
medication, 106, 109
skills training, 106–107, 260, 263
therapeutic alliance, 103–105,
    108, 109, 154–155
*Psychiatric Rehabilitation of Chronic
    Mental Patients*, 241, 244, 247,
    251
Psychoanalytic theories
    contemporary treatment
        perspective, 14–17
    historical perspective, 9–11
Psychoeducational interventions,
    129
Psychosocial rehabilitation, 129

Research issues
    adversarial attitude of clinicians,
        136–137
    attribution theory, 137–138
    clinician's behavior as stressor,
        131–138, 164–165
    coping strategies of families,
        149–153, 164
    cross-cultural, 140, 142–144
    defense strategies, 136
    deinstitutionalization, family role
        in, 145–147
    ethical issues, 147–149
    expressed emotion, 144–145
    families of mentally ill, 164–165
    family deviance, 138–140
    need for new therapeutic models,
        153–154
    professional-family therapeutic
        alliances, 154–155
    schizophrenia, 220–221
    stressful life events, 129–131
    stress-vulnerability-protective
        framework, 263–264
Resistant family members, 180,
    182–184
Responsibility for care of mentally
    ill, 78–80

Retribution for family
    noncompliance, 181–182, 185

Schizophrenia
    biological roots, 118
    clinical failures, 219–220
    cross-cultural studies, 142–143
    education of family, 105–106
    education of mental health
        professionals, 165–168
    and expressed emotion, 23–24,
        142–143, 274
    family deviance, 139–140
    family influence, 15, 26–29
    historical perspective, 10, 13
    impact on children, 41–42
    impact on family, 35–36,
        163–164, 259–260, 262
    impact on siblings, 40–41, 150,
        262
    individual therapy for, 128–129
    model of illness, 167–168
    treatment approach, 165–167
Secondary disability, 93–94
Shaw v. Glickman, 177
Siblings of the mentally ill, 40–41,
    150, 262
Social Behavior Assessment
    Schedule, 270
Social disablement. *See* Tertiary
    disability
Social pressure and disability
    relationship, 94–95
Social protest, 81–82
Social work, unpopularity, 224
Spouses of the mentally ill, 40
Stress factors
    assessment, 269–272
    patient-relatedness, 268, 270–271
    for relatives, 257–258, 259–260,
        262, 268
    research issues, 164
Stress management, 107, 260–261,
    272–275
Stress-vulnerability-protective
    framework
    critique, 268
    described, 256–257
    outcomes for relatives, 262
    prodromes of dysfunction in
        relatives, 261
    provider-family relationship, 263

relatives of the mentally ill,
257–261
research issues, 263–264
Subjective burden of mental illness,
37–38, 271–272
Support networks, 45–46, 56, 261

Tertiary disability, 94
Thorazine. *See* Chlorpromazine

UCLA curriculum
evaluation, 251–252
goals, 244–247
instruction methods, 247–251
obstacles, 242–244
UCLA Family Project, 15–16
University of Wisconsin-Madison
School of Social Work
curriculum
agency benefits, 226–227

attitudes of students, 225–226
competencies after one year,
237–238
goals, 227–228
instruction methods, 228–230
obstacles, 224–226
other assignments, 232–235
placements, 230–231
reading and writing assignments,
231–232
student development, 235–237

Vulnerability factors
of patients, 256
of relatives, 257, 258–259, 262

"Worried well patients," 116–117